Contents

Cardiovascular disease prevention

David Wood MSc, FRCP, FRCPE, FFPHM, FESC
Garfield Weston Professor of Cardiovascular Medicine
National Heart and Lung Institute
Imperial College
London, UK

Kornelia Kotseva MD, PhD, FESC
Senior Clinical Research Fellow
Cardiovascular Medicine
National Heart and Lung Institute
Imperial College
London, UK

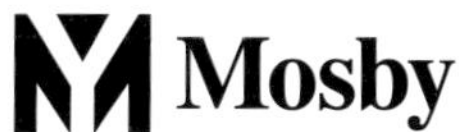
Mosby

MOSBY
An imprint of Elsevier Limited.

The Publisher's policy is to use **paper manufactured from sustainable forests**

Mosby is a registered trademark of Elsevier Limited.

ISBN 0-7234-3358-5

Cataloguing in Publication Data
Catalogue records for this book are available from the US Library of Congress and the British Library.

Note
Medical knowledge is constantly changing. As new information becomes available, changes in treatment, procedures, equipment and the use of drugs become necessary. The editors/authors/contributors and the publishers have taken care to ensure that the information given in this text is accurate and up to date. However, readers are strongly advised to confirm that the information, especially with regard to drug usage, complies with the latest legislation and standards of practice.

Printed in China.

Foreword

Prevention of atherosclerotic cardiovascular diseases is part of modern every day clinical practice in both hospital and primary care. This rapid reference provides focussed practical guidance on lifestyle and risk factor management, including drug treatments, for patients with established atherosclerotic disease and apparently healthy individuals at high risk of developing this disease. The text is drawn primarily from the Joint European Societies guidance on coronary and cardiovascular disease prevention between 1994 and 2003, the Joint British Societies recommendations on coronary heart disease prevention in 1998 and the most recent professional guidelines from the United States on hypertension, lipids and diabetes. The scientific evidence that modifying lifestyle and other risk factors, and prescribing cardioprotective drug therapies will reduce cardiovascular morbidity and mortality is compelling. The clinical challenge is to translate this evidence into effective clinical care.

David Wood and Kornelia Kotseva

Introduction and background

Cardiovascular diseases (CVD), of which coronary heart disease (CHD) is the most common, are the major causes of death in middle-aged and older patients in most developed countries and in many developing countries. Cardiovascular diseases result in substantial disability worldwide and contribute in large part to the escalating costs of healthcare, especially with an increasing ageing population. Currently, CHD is predicted to be the leading cause of death and disability-adjusted life years by 2020.[1,2] This is largely because of an increasing burden of CVD in developing countries.

Cardiovascular disease mortality

According to the World Health Organization over the period 1965–1998, CVD mortality rate has been declining substantially in North America since the early 1970s and in most Western European countries since the late 1970s, but with major geographical differences between countries.[3]

In the USA the long-term trends in CHD mortality are favourable with an age-standardized mortality rate of around 121/100,000 for men and 67/100,000 for women in 1995–1997.

In the whole European Union, age-standardized CHD mortality rate in men rose from around 146/100,000 in 1965–1969 to around 159/100,000 in 1975–1979, and declined thereafter by 32% to around 99/100,000 in 1995–1998. In women, the pattern was similar, with a peak at around 68/100,000 women in 1975–1979 and a subsequent decline by 30% to around 44/100,000 women in 1995–1997.

Although major geographical differences in CHD mortality persisted within Western Europe (185/100,000 men in Ireland *vs* 49/100,000 men in France), and mortality rate decreases were greater in some countries (Finland and the Netherlands) than others (Germany, Ireland and Portugal), the declines were steady within geographical areas and countries.

In contrast in Eastern Europe, CHD mortality tended to rise until the early 1990s but has declined over the past few years in Poland and the Czech Republic. In the Russian Federation, mortality rates from CHD reached 330/100,000 men and 154/100,000 women during 1995–1998. The highest mortality rates in 1995–1998 were registered in Ukraine, reaching around 394/100,000 men and 223/100,000 women.

Figures 1 and 2 show the histograms of CHD in 49 countries (or groups of countries) based on the most recent available data (period 1995–1998). CHD mortality rates are highest in Eastern European countries, with an almost 10-fold difference between countries with the highest mortality rates and those with the lowest mortality rates.

Japan, an industrialized nation, provides an interesting comparator for CHD mortality with other economically developed countries. The CHD mortality rate was already low in the late 1960s and then declined further to 36/100,000 for men and 17/100,000 for women in 1995–1997; one of the lowest official CHD mortality rates worldwide.

Pathogenesis of atherosclerosis

The normal artery

The normal artery consists of an intima, a media and an adventitia. The intima is lined by endothelial cells on the inner (luminal) aspect of the vessel, and is bounded by the internal elastic lamina on its outer aspect. These cells form a continuous, smooth, uninterrupted surface, and represent the principal barrier between blood and the arterial wall. They have nonthrombogenic properties, and are capable of metabolizing numerous vasoactive substances, such a prostacyclin (PGI2) and nitric oxide, and of producing growth factors and forming connective tissue matrix. They can also interact with platelets, monocytes, T-lymphocytes and smooth muscle cells.

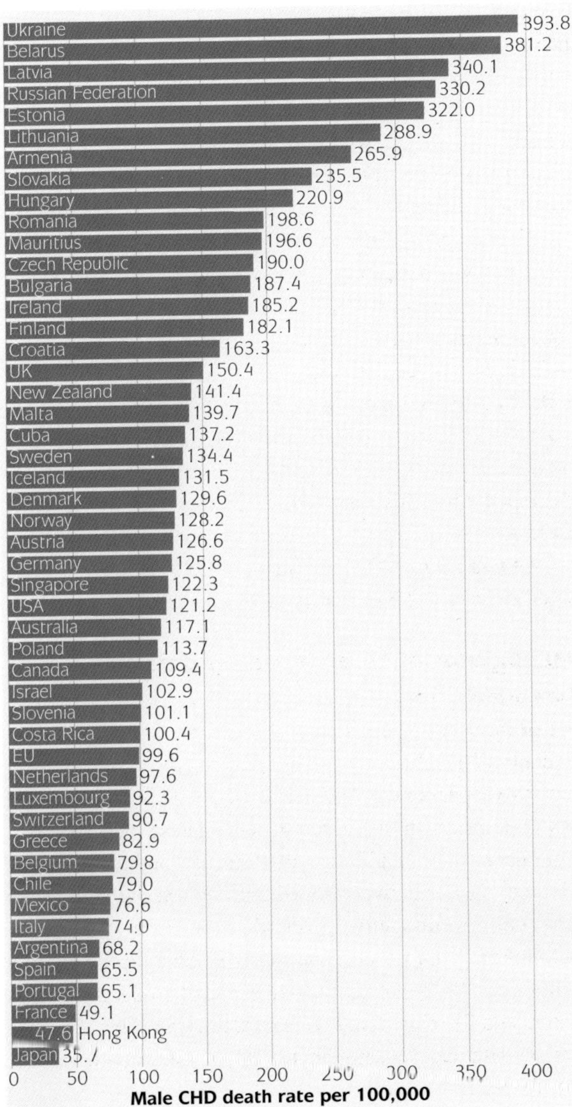

Figure 1. Age-standardized death certification rates from coronary heart diseases in men in 48 countries and the European Union, 1995–1998. Reproduced with permission from Levi F *et al*. *Heart* 2002;**88**:119–124.

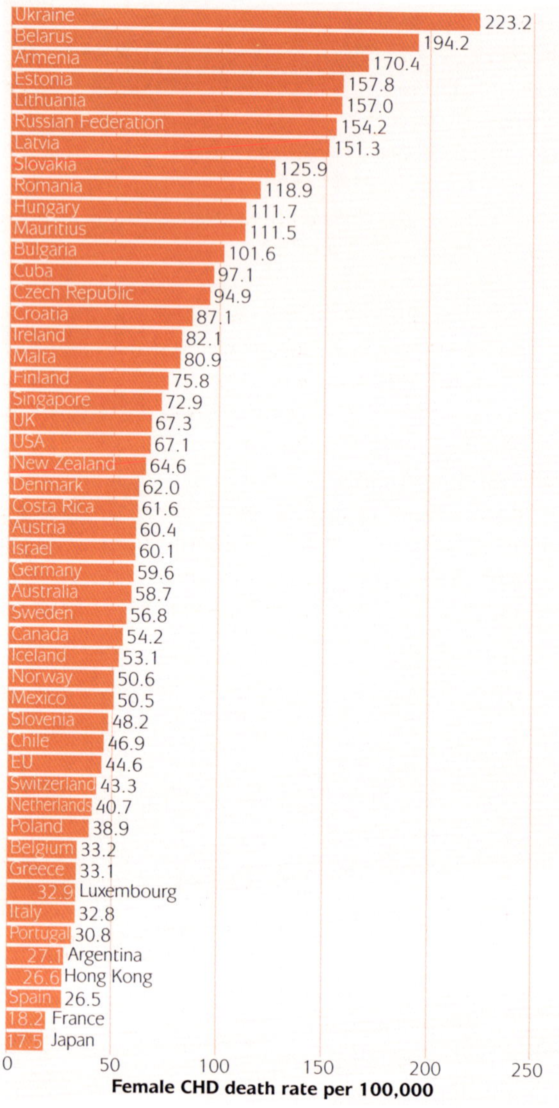

Figure 2. Age-standardized death certification rates from coronary heart diseases in women in 48 countries and the European Union, 1995–1998. Reproduced with permission from Levi F *et al*. *Heart* 2002;**88**:119–124.

Pathology of atherosclerosis

Atherosclerosis is a progressive disease that can begin in early life and usually becomes clinically manifest in middle-to-late adulthood. The earliest lesion of atherosclerosis, called a fatty streak, has been found in young children. The advanced lesion of atherosclerosis is a lipid-rich fibrous plaque (Figure 3).

This is the result of three fundamental biological processes, which are described in Table 1.

Clinical expressions of atherosclerosis

Atherosclerosis principally affects medium-sized muscular arteries, including the coronary, carotid, basilar and vertebral arteries, as well as the arteries of lower extremities, in particular the iliac and superficial femoral arteries. Larger arteries, such as the aorta and others, can also be involved. The main clinical manifestations of atherosclerosis are coronary, cerebral and peripheral arterial diseases. Acute expansion of the atherosclerotic lesion occurs when the endothelial cells rupture, allowing haemorrhage into the

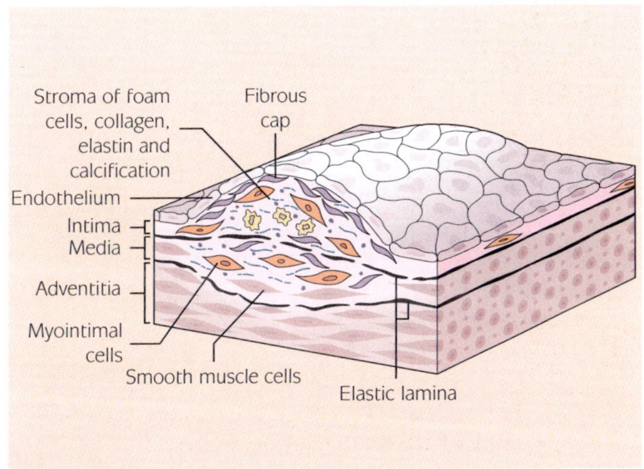

Figure 3. Diagrammatic representation of a cross-section of a fibrous plaque. Reproduced with permission from *Lipids, Diabetes and Vascular Disease (second edition)*. Dodson PM, Barnett AH (eds). London: Science Press Ltd, 1998.

Formation of an advanced atherosclerotic lesion
The advanced lesion of atherosclerosis is the result of three fundamental biological processes: 1. Accumulation of intimal smooth muscle cells, together with variable numbers of accumulated macrophages and T-lymphocytes 2. Formation by the proliferated smooth muscle cells of large amounts of connective tissue matrix, including collagen, elastic fibres and proteoglycans 3. Accumulation of lipid, principally in the form of cholesteryl esters, and free cholesterol within the cells and in the surrounding connective tissues

Table 1. The three fundamental biological processes involved in the formation of an advanced lesion of atherosclerosis.

plaque and platelet aggregation on the endothelial surface. When plaque rupture occurs and thrombogenic substances are exposed, the arterial lumen may become obstructed by a combination of fibrin, platelet aggregates and red blood cells. Plaque rupture is now considered to be the common pathophysiological substrate of the acute ischaemic syndromes, which, in coronary arteries, range from unstable angina through to Q-wave acute myocardial infarction.

Risk factors for atherosclerotic diseases

Definition of a risk factor

Epidemiological, clinical and basic research over the past five decades has provided considerable knowledge about the causes and natural history of CVD. Environmental and lifestyle characteristics, and physiological, biochemical, genetic and other factors have been related to the development of CVD. They are known as *risk factors*, a term which describes those characteristics found in healthy individuals to be independently related to the subsequent occurrence of CVD and, where modifiable, to be reversible. These risk factors are aetiologically related to the development of CVD, and their modification can prevent the development of the disease. When a person develops symptomatic CHD or other atherosclerotic disease, the modifiable risk factors continue to contribute to disease progression and prognosis.

There is a wealth of epidemiological, clinical and basic scientific evidence that lifestyle risk factors – a diet rich in saturated fats and calories, smoking and physical inactivity – have an important role in causing and contributing to the development of CVD. These lifestyle risk factors lead, in many individuals, to adverse changes in physiological and biochemical characteristics, such as blood pressure, plasma lipids and glycaemia, which encourage the development of atherosclerosis and associated thrombotic complications (*see* Table 2). There can also be a genetic component in the susceptibility of individuals to atherosclerotic CVD.

Epidemiology of risk factors and the development of atherosclerotic disease

Lifestyle

Smoking

Smoking increases the risk of developing cardiovascular disease, and is responsible for 50% of all avoidable deaths,

Lifestyle and characteristics associated with increased risk of cardiovascular diseases	
Lifestyles	• Diet high in saturated fat, cholesterol and calories • Tobacco smoking • Excess alcohol consumption • Physical inactivity • Obesity
Biochemical or physiological characteristics (modifiable)	• Elevated blood pressure • Elevated plasma total cholesterol (LDL-cholesterol) • Low plasma HDL-cholesterol • Elevated plasma triglycerides • Elevated plasma glucose/diabetes • Thrombogenic factors
Personal characteristics (non-modifiable)	• Age • Sex • Family history of CHD or other atherosclerotic vascular disease at early age (men <55, women <65) • Personal history of CHD or other atherosclerotic vascular disease

Table 2. Lifestyle and characteristics associated with an increased risk of future coronary heart disease events. Reproduced with permission from Wood D *et al. Eur Heart J* 1998;**19**:1434–1503.

half of which are due to CVD.[4,5] This adverse effect of smoking is related to the amount of tobacco smoked daily and the duration of smoking. The risk of future CVD is particularly high if smoking starts before the age of 15 years. Passive smoking has now been shown to increase the risk of CHD and other smoking- related diseases for example, lung cancer. [6-8]

Diet

Diet is an important determinant of CVD risk.[9-11] A diet high in saturated and *trans* fatty acids, and cholesterol increases the risk of CVD. The effect of diet on the development of atherosclerosis is mediated through the influence of other risk factors such as blood pressure, low-density lipoprotein (LDL), high-density lipoprotein (HDL), glycaemia and the propensity to thrombosis.

Physical inactivity

A sedentary lifestyle increases the risk of death from all causes and CVD.[12-17]

Obesity

Obesity is a consequence of a diet high in calories (usually from saturated fat) and physical inactivity. It is associated with an increase in all-cause and cardiovascular mortality, and has an adverse effect on cardiovascular risk factors such as high blood pressure, elevated plasma LDL-cholesterol and HDL-cholesterol, increased triglycerides and glucose intolerance.[18] Central adiposity, with an increased intra-abdominal fat mass, is associated with a particularly adverse profile of these risk factors and also with insulin resistance (*see Glycaemia and diabetes*). It is more strongly associated with the risk of CHD and other CVD than general adiposity, as assessed by the body mass index (BMI).[19-21] The risk of CHD already begins to increase at moderate levels of weight gain and overweight. Overweight is also associated with an increased risk of stroke.

Alcohol

Moderate alcohol intake is associated with lower risk of CHD.[22] Alcohol increases plasma HDL-cholesterol level, and this may partly explain the cardioprotective effect of alcohol. It has also been shown that alcohol has an anti-aggregatory effect on platelets and a favourable effect on fibrinolytic factors. However, increasing alcohol consumption has been associated with an increased prevalence of hypertension and increased risk of haemorrhagic stroke. Furthermore, heavy drinking increases the risk of sudden arrhythmic death. At an individual level, where there are no contra-indications to alcohol use, 10–30 g of ethanol per day for men and 10–20 g of ethanol per day for women may be considered safe.[23]

Physiological and biochemical risk factors

Blood pressure

As systolic and diastolic blood pressures (SBP and DBP) increase, so does the risk of CHD, heart failure, cerebrovascular disease and renal failure in both men and women.[24-26] Following myocardial infarction (MI), blood pressure elevation is associated with an increased risk of re-infarction and coronary death, as well as an increased risk of stroke. SBP is an independent and strong predictor of risk of cardiovascular and renal disease. Elevated SBP is a major risk factor in the elderly.

Lipids

Lipids are also important risk factors for CVD. The degree to which lipoproteins cause atherosclerosis depends in part on their size. The smallest lipoproteins, HDL, enter the artery wall, and also leave it, easily, and do not cause atherosclerosis. In contrast, LDL, intermediate density lipoproteins (IDL) and small species of very low density lipoproteins (VLDL) are small enough to enter the artery wall, and, if chemically modified by oxidation, are easily retained in the wall to cause atherosclerosis. The largest lipoproteins, chylomicrons and large VLDL, are too large to enter the artery wall, and are therefore not atherogenic.

LDL-cholesterol

As total plasma cholesterol (or LDL-cholesterol) increases, so does the risk of CVD.[27-29] This relationship applies to both healthy individuals and to patients with established CHD. The relationship between total or LDL-cholesterol and CVD is modified by other lipid factors. Low HDL-cholesterol and raised triglycerides increase the risk of any level of LDL-cholesterol. In patients with the heterozygous form of familial hypercholesterolemia, LDL-cholesterol can be quite elevated (7–12 mmol/l, 270–465 mg/dl) and extremely elevated in the rare homozygous form (12–20 mmol/l, 465–770 mg/dl). In this latter case, LDL-cholesterol causes aggressive CHD in early life even if there are no other risk factors.

Triglycerides

As triglycerides increase, so does the risk of CHD; however, this association is not as strong as it is for LDL-cholesterol. Triglycerides up to 5 mmol/l (about 450 mg/dl) predict the risk of CHD, and this relationship is stronger in women and younger individuals.[30-32]

HDL-cholesterol

As plasma HDL-cholesterol decreases, the risk of CHD increases.[33] This inverse relationship has been shown for both men and women, in healthy individuals and patients with CHD.

A combination of plasma triglycerides higher than 2 mmol/l (180 mg/dl) and HDL-cholesterol lower than 1 mmol/l (40 mg/dl) predicts a high risk of CHD, especially if the ratio of cholesterol:HDL cholesterol is greater than 5.

Glycaemia and diabetes

As non-fasting glucose levels increase so does the risk of CVD. This has been shown in individuals without diabetes using the 2-hour glucose value, following an oral glucose-tolerance test, or the glycated haemoglobin (HbA1c) concentration.[34] Impaired glucose tolerance (IGT) – the intermediate stage between normal and diabetic post-load glucose levels – and diabetes are also associated with an increase in risk of CVD.[35]

In Type 1 (insulin-dependent) diabetes, there is a two- to three-fold increase in risk of developing CVD, CHD and stroke, but this risk is almost entirely confined to those patients developing diabetic renal disease. In Type 2 (non-insulin-dependent) diabetes, all patients are at increased risk of CVD, even in the absence of diabetic nephropathy.

Type 2 diabetes is associated with an abnormal cardiovascular risk profile. Even at the precursor stage of Type 2 diabetes, in which IGT is diagnosed by an oral glucose tolerance test, the cardiovascular risk factor pattern is characteristic of Type 2 diabetes – central type of obesity, elevated plasma triglycerides and low plasma HDL-cholesterol, elevated blood pressure and hyperinsulinaemia, which reflects insulin resistance of the peripheral tissues, in particular skeletal muscles. This adverse pattern of cardiovascular risk factors, which may last for many years in the IGT phase progressing towards diabetes, explains why many patients at the time of diagnosis of Type 2 diabetes, already have clinically manifest CVD.

Glucose regulation can be classified on fasting and 2-hour plasma glucose levels (following a 75-g oral glucose load) into:[36-40]

- Normal glucose tolerance
- Impaired fasting glycaemia
- Impaired glucose tolerance
- Diabetes mellitus.

This classification of glycaemia by the oral glucose tolerance test is shown in Table 3.

Insulin resistance

Hyperinsulinaemia is associated with several cardiovascular risk factors (*see* Table 4).[41,42] Individuals with this cluster of risk factors have a decreased sensitivity of peripheral tissues, in particular skeletal muscles, to the action of insulin. This is

Classification of glycaemia		
	Fasting plasma glucose	**2-hour plasma glucose**
Normal	≤ 6.0 mmol/l	< 7.8 mmol/l
Impaired fasting glycaemia	6.1–6.9 mmol/l	< 7.8 mmol/l
Impaired glucose tolerance	< 7.0 mmol/l	7.8–11.0 mmol/l
Diabetes	≥ 7.0 mmol/l	≥ 11.1 mmol/l

Table 3. Classification of glycaemia by the oral glucose tolerance test.

termed the *insulin resistance syndrome* or, more commonly, the *metabolic syndrome* (*see* Table 5). Individuals with this syndrome have an increased risk of developing Type 2 diabetes, and are at increased risk of CVD even if they do not develop diabetes.[43]

Risk factors associated with insulin resistance

Cardiovascular risk factors that are associated with hyperinsulinaemia include:

- Central obesity
- Elevated blood pressure
- Elevated plasma triglycerides
- Low HDL-cholesterol
- Impaired glucose tolerance

Table 4. Cardiovascular risk factors associated with hyperinsulinaemia and insulin resistance.

Clinical identification of the metabolic syndrome

Risk factor	**Defining level**
Abdominal obesity	Waist circumference
Men	>102cm (> 40in)
Women	> 88cm (>35in)
Triglycerides	≥ 150mg/dl
HDL-cholesterol	
Men	< 40mg/dl
Women	< 50mg/dl
Blood pressure	≥ 130/85mmHg
Fasting glucose	≥ 110mg/dl

Table 5. Clinical identification of the metabolic syndrome. Abdominal obesity is a key risk factor. Reproduced with permission from National Cholesterol Education Program, National Institutes of Health, NIH Publication No. 01-3670, May 2001.

Other risk factors

Raised plasma homocysteine (tHcy) is associated with increased risk of CHD.[44] The components and factors of coagulation and fibrinolysis, including fibrinogen, C-reactive protein, albumin, white cell count, haematocrit, viscosity and erythrocyte sedimentation rate, have all been associated with an increase in risk of cardiovascular events. Other markers for the development of CVD include von Willebrand factor, D-dimer antigen, Factor VII and plasminogen levels.

Inflammatory processes may also have a role in the pathogenesis of atherosclerosis and the development of CVD.[45] Elevations of plasma C-reactive protein, a marker of inflammation, predict the risk of developing CHD events, stroke and peripheral vascular disease in healthy individuals, and the risk of CHD events in patients with unstable and stable angina pectoris. The association between elevated plasma fibrinogen and CHD risk may also, in part, reflect an on-going inflammatory process because fibrinogen is an acute-phase reactant.

Chronic infections with micro-organisms, such as *Chlamydia pneumoniae* and *Helicobacter pylori*, and cytomegalovirus may be related to the development of CVD.[46] However, evidence is conflicting and the sequence of infection, development of atherosclerotic lesions and plaque rupture still remains uncertain.

Genetics

Family history

Family history of CHD is a risk factor for CVD (Table 6).[47] A detailed family history of CHD, or other atherosclerotic disease, should be part of the assessment of all patients with CHD for the identification of high-risk individuals.

A family history of premature CHD should also be taken into account in assessing the risk of a healthy individual developing CVD. Lifestyle advice and, where appropriate, therapeutic management of risk factors should be offered to members of families where coronary disease, or other atherosclerotic disease, occurs prematurely or is particularly prevalent.

Familial hypercholesterolemia is a monogenic disorder, caused by mutations of the LDL-receptor gene, resulting in very high levels of cholesterol, (usually a total cholesterol > 8 mmol/l; > 300 mg/dl) with an LDL cholesterol higher than 6.0 mmol/l (240 mg/dl) and often family history of premature CHD. Familial hypercholesterolaemia is associated with a very high risk of premature CHD. High blood cholesterol in an individual, especially if there is a family history of premature CHD, should lead to systematic screening of all the close relatives.

Family history and risk of CHD

The risk of CHD increases:

- When an individual is closely related to a family member who has developed CHD (i.e. in first-degree relatives – siblings and offspring)
- As the percentage of family members with CHD increases; and
- The younger the age at which family members develop CHD. Risk factor screening should be considered in the first-degree relatives of patients with premature CHD (< 55 years in men and < 65 years in women)

Table 6. Family history factors increasing the risk of CHD.

Assessment of cardiovascular risk

Concept of absolute multifactorial risk

Absolute risk of CVD is the probability of an individual developing the disease over a defined period (e.g. within the next 10 years).

As CVD is multifactorial in its origins, it is important, in estimating the risk of developing or having recurrent CVD, to consider all risk factors simultaneously. Traditionally, risk factor guidelines have been concerned with unifactorial assessment (e.g. in the management of hypertension, dyslipidaemia or diabetes), and this has resulted in undue emphasis being placed on individually high risk factors rather than the overall level of risk based on all factors taken together. In practice, physicians deal with the whole patient rather than one aspect of his or her risk. In addition, clustering of risk factors in an individual may have a multiplicative effect on absolute disease risk. Therefore, an individual with a number of mildly abnormal risk factors may be at greater absolute CVD risk than a subject with just one high risk factor (Table 7).

Patients with symptomatic atherosclerosis

Patients with clinically manifest CVD are at very high absolute risk of a further vascular event. It is not necessary to risk stratify these patients because they all require the most intensive lifestyle interventions and drug therapies to achieve risk factor goals and protect the vasculature. Patients with clinically established CVD have, at any level of a single risk factor or any combination of risk factors, a much higher risk of recurrent disease than asymptomatic persons. As modifiable risk factors continue to influence the subsequent risk of CVD events in patients with clinically established CVD, it is important to address all risk factors in the care of such patients.

Absolute risk of developing a CHD event						
Sex	**Age (years)**	**Plasma cholesterol (mmol/l)**	**Systolic blood pressure (mmHg)**	**Smoking**	**Clinical CHD**	**Minimum estimate of 10-year risk**
Male	50	7	120	–	–	10%
Male	50	6	140	+	–	20%
Male	50	7	120	–	+	>20%
Male	50	6	140	+	+	>40%

Table 7. Examples showing the impact of a single risk factor, multiple risk factors and clinically established CHD on the absolute risk of developing a CHD event over 10 years. Reproduced with permission from Wood D *et al. Eur Heart J* 1998;**19**:1434–1503.

Healthy individuals and absolute multifactorial risk assessment

In apparently healthy individuals it is important to estimate absolute CHD or CVD risk by taking into account all the major risk factors. Those at highest multifactorial risk can be identified and targeted for lifestyle interventions and, where appropriate, drug therapies. Physicians should always use absolute disease risk when making a clinical judgement about using drugs to treat blood pressure and blood lipids, rather than just considering the level of any one risk factor alone.

The advantages of a multifactorial approach to treatment of high-risk individuals are listed in Table 8.

The disadvantage of a multifactorial approach to primary prevention of CVD is that treatment is concentrated on the older population unless the effect of lifetime exposure to risk factors is taken into account.

Cardiovascular disease risk based on the Framingham study

Calculation of coronary or cardiovascular risk is now widely advocated in international and national guidelines for CVD prevention. Practical methods – charts, tables and computer

Advantages of a multifactorial approach to the treatment of high-risk individuals

- Concept of continuous risk replaces the traditional dichotomous classification of risk factors
- Level of absolute (multifactorial) risk for which treatment is given is not fixed
- Treatment is targeted at those with the highest absolute CVD risk
- Benefit is greatest in those at highest multifactorial risk
- Avoiding treatment of single risk factors in those at low multifactorial risk

Table 8. Advantages of a multifactorial approach to the treatment of high-risk individuals.

programmes – have been developed for assessing an individual's absolute risk of developing CVD on the basis of risk functions derived from prospective epidemiological studies. The majority of these methods are based on the risk function derived from the Framingham study,[48] which forms the basis of the risk charts and assessment tools in New Zealand, Europe, the UK and USA.[49-59]

Cardiovascular risk prediction in Europe

The calculation of total CHD risk for healthy individuals was advocated in the European recommendations on coronary prevention in 1994 and 1998, and a simplified method of deriving an approximate 10-year CHD risk based on Framingham was presented in the form of a coronary risk chart (Figures 4 and 5).[52,53] An individual's absolute risk of developing a CHD event (angina, non-fatal MI or coronary death) over the next 10 years is found by locating the appropriate box in the charts in relation to the patient's age, gender, smoking status, blood pressure and cholesterol levels. A separate risk chart was produced for patients with diabetes mellitus (Figures 6 and 7).

The 10-year CHD risk is presented in five levels:

- low (< 5%)
- mild (5–10%)
- moderate (10–20%)
- high (20–40%)
- very high (> 40%).

An absolute risk of 20% or more was defined as the threshold for intensive risk factor intervention. An absolute risk that exceeds 20% over the next 10 years, or will exceed 20% if projected to age 60, and is sustained despite professional lifestyle intervention, was considered to be sufficiently high to justify the selective use of proven drug therapies.

Certain individuals are at higher risk than is evident from the coronary risk chart. Risk is higher than indicated in patients with familial dyslipidaemias, family history of premature CVD, low HDL-cholesterol or raised triglyceride levels, and other risk factors. With these caveats the chart performs several functions:

- An individual's absolute risk of developing a CHD event in the next decade, or when projected to age 60 years, can be read from the chart without any calculations.
- Relative risk can be estimated by comparing the risk in one cell with any other in the same age group.
- The chart can be used to show the potential effect of changing from one risk category to another by stopping smoking, reducing blood pressure or total cholesterol.
- Although young people are at lower risk than older people, risk rises steadily with increasing age. The chart can be used to illustrate the effect of lifetime risk, by following the boxes upwards and observing the increasing risk with increasing age if risk factors remain constant.

CHD risk prediction based on Framingham is now being replaced in Europe by a new European risk function called SCORE as advocated in the most recent European guidelines on CVD prevention published in 2003.

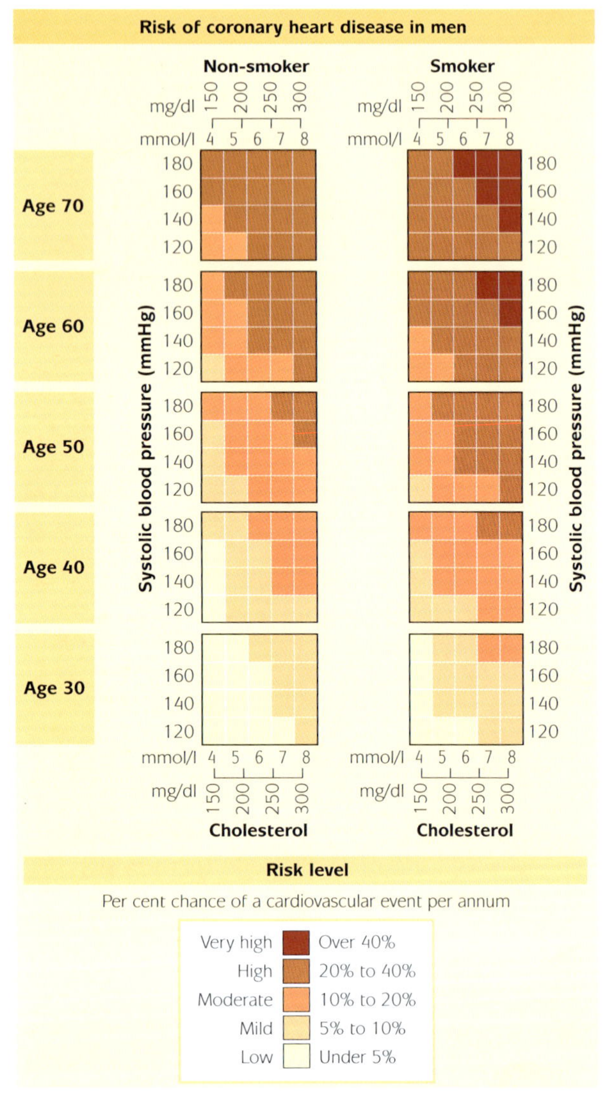

Figure 4. Coronary risk chart for primary CHD prevention in men. Reproduced with permission from Wood D *et al.* *Eur Heart J* 1998;**19**:1434–1503.

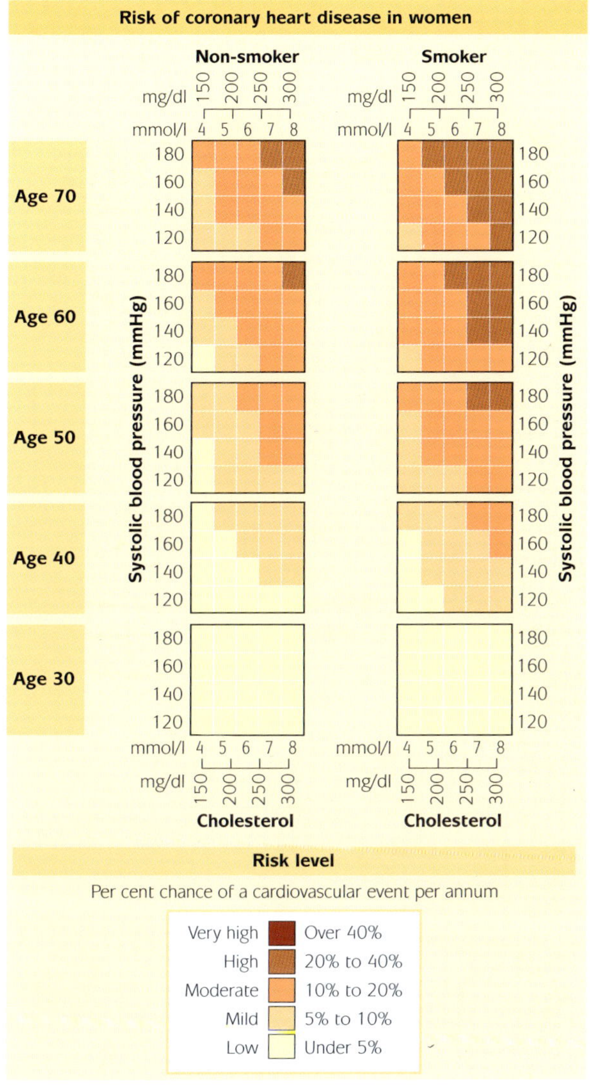

Figure 5. Coronary risk chart for primary CHD prevention in women. Reproduced with permission from Wood D *et al.* *Eur Heart J* 1998;**19**:1434–1503.

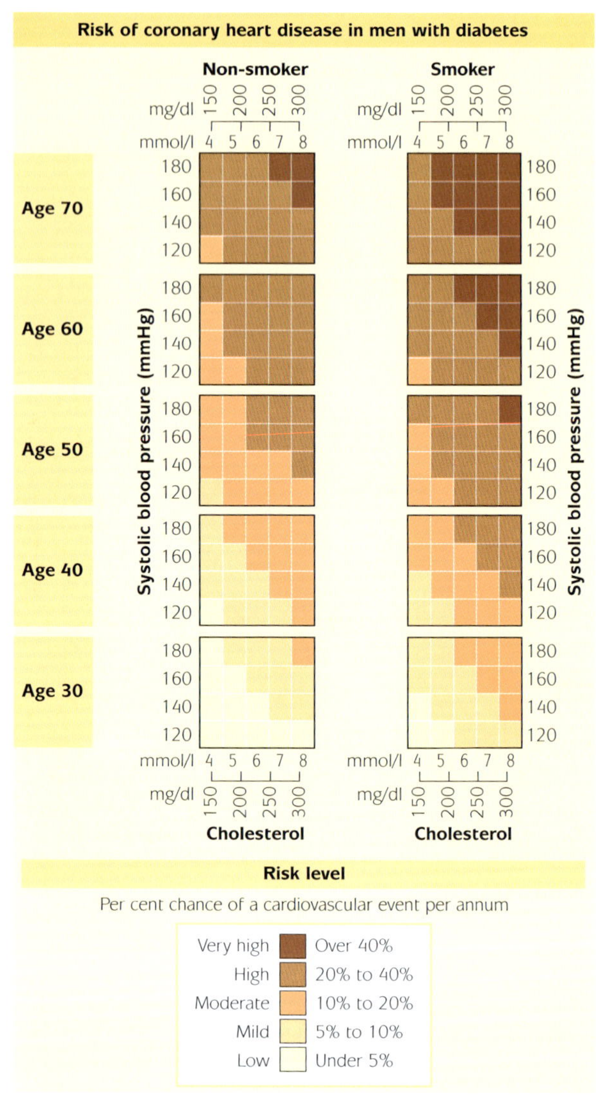

Figure 6. Coronary risk chart for primary CHD prevention in men with diabetes. Reproduced with permission from Wood D *et al. Eur Heart J* 1998;**19**:1434–1503.

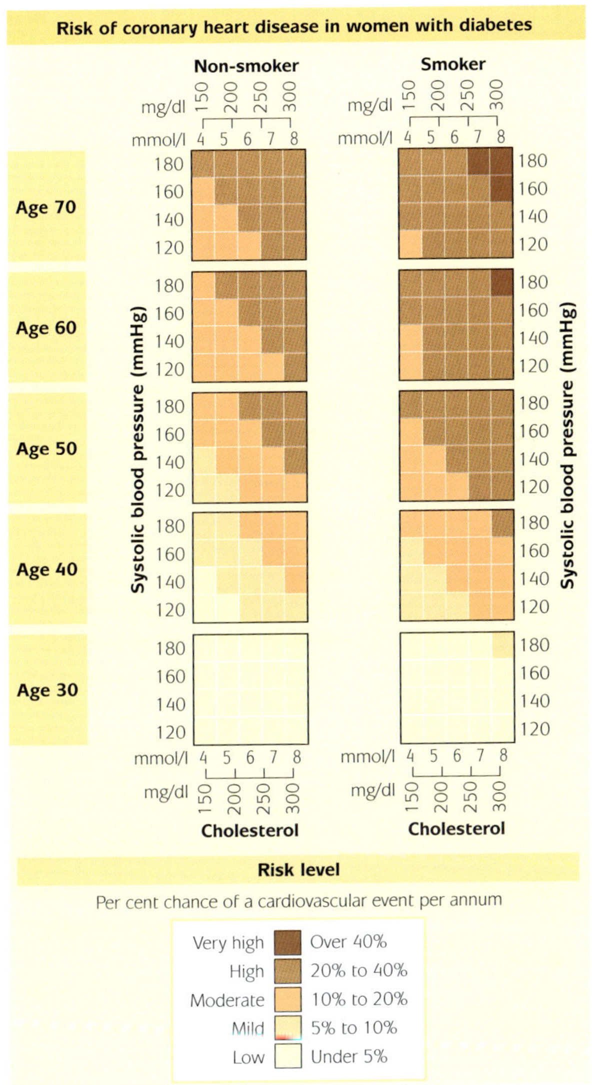

Figure 7. Coronary risk chart for primary CHD prevention in women with diabetes. Reproduced with permission from Wood D *et al. Eur Heart J* 1998;**19**:1434–1503.

Cardiovascular risk prediction in the UK

The Joint British Societies produced a coronary risk prediction chart and an associated computer programme "Cardiac Risk Assessor" based on Framingham.[55,56] The latter calculates both 10-year CHD and CVD risks (including stroke) over the same period. The British chart is based on age, sex, smoking, systolic blood pressure and the ratio total cholesterol:HDL-cholesterol (Figure 8). A separate chart was produced for patients with diabetes mellitus (Figure 9).

The projected 10-year CHD risk is represented graphically as a function of systolic blood pressure (110–220 mmHg) on the vertical axis, and the cholesterol:HDL ratio (3–12) on the horizontal axis. CHD risk is classified in three categories: < 15%; 15–30% and > 30%. High-risk individuals are defined as those whose 10-year risk of CHD exceeds 15% (equivalent to a cardiovascular risk of 20% over the same period) or will exceed 15% if projected to age 60 years. It was recommended that, as a minimum, those at highest risk (≥ 30%) should be targeted and treated straight away and, as resources allowed, others with a risk greater than 15% should be progressively targeted.

Cardiovascular risk prediction in the USA

The Third Report of the Expert Panel on Detection, Evaluation, and Treatment of High Blood Cholesterol in Adults (known as Adult Treatment Panel III or ATP III) also advocated the multiple risk factor approach for identification and treatment of high-risk individuals.[59] The Framingham projections of 10-year absolute CHD risk are used to identify patients with multiple risk factors for more intensive treatment. Lowering of LDL-cholesterol is the primary goal of therapy and there are three categories of risk for different LDL goals and different intensities of LDL-lowering therapy (Table 9):

1. The highest risk category consists of CHD and CHD equivalents (other forms of clinical atherosclerotic disease), which carry a risk for major coronary events greater than 20% per 10 years. The LDL goal is less than 100 mg/dl.

2. The second risk category comprises people with multiple (two or more) risk factors (smoking, hypertension, low HDL-cholesterol, family history of premature CHD, age [male ≥ 45 years and female ≥ 55 years] and diabetes) and 10-year risk for CHD no greater than 20%. The LDL goal is less than 130 mg/dl.
3. The third risk category includes people who have no more than one risk factor, 10-year risk for CHD less than 10%. The LDL goal is less than 160 mg/dl.

Risk status in people without clinically manifest CHD or other forms of atherosclerotic disease is determined by a two-step procedure. First, the number of risk factors is counted. Second, for people with multiple (two or more) risk factors, 10-year risk assessment is carried out with the Framingham scoring system to identify individuals whose risk warrants intensive treatment (Tables 10 and 11).

When no more than one risk factor is present, the Framingham scoring system is not necessary because 10-year risk rarely reaches the level for intensive treatment. Risk factors used in Framingham scoring include age, total cholesterol, HDL-cholesterol, blood pressure and cigarette smoking. The first step is to calculate the number of points for each risk factor and the total risk score. The 10-year risk for MI and coronary death is derived from this total score, and the person is categorized according to absolute 10-year CHD risk. The Framingham scoring system divides people with multiple risk factors according to 10-year CHD risk: less than 10%, between 10 and 20%, or greater than 20%.

Cardiovascular risk based on the European SCORE project

A European risk function called SCORE has been developed because Framingham has certain limitations. First, the Framingham Heart Study is based on only 5,573 individuals and, despite the long period of follow-up, risk estimation in younger age groups, especially in women, is not based on sufficient cardiovascular events. Second, the risk function derived from a high-risk middle-aged North American

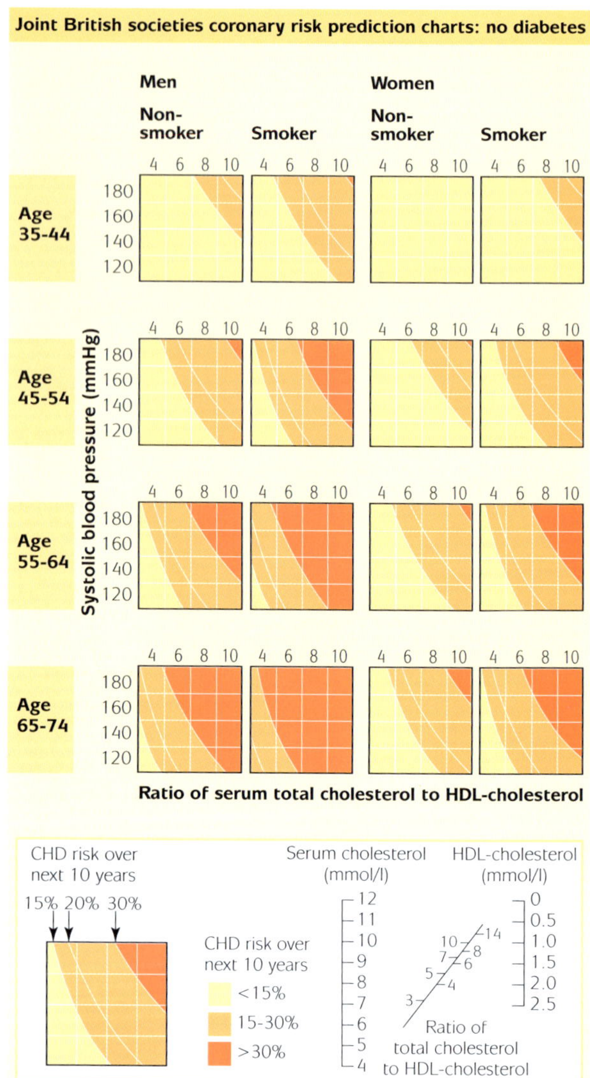

Figure 8. Joint British societies coronary risk prediction charts for people without diabetes. Reproduced with permission from *BMJ* 2000;**320**:705–708.

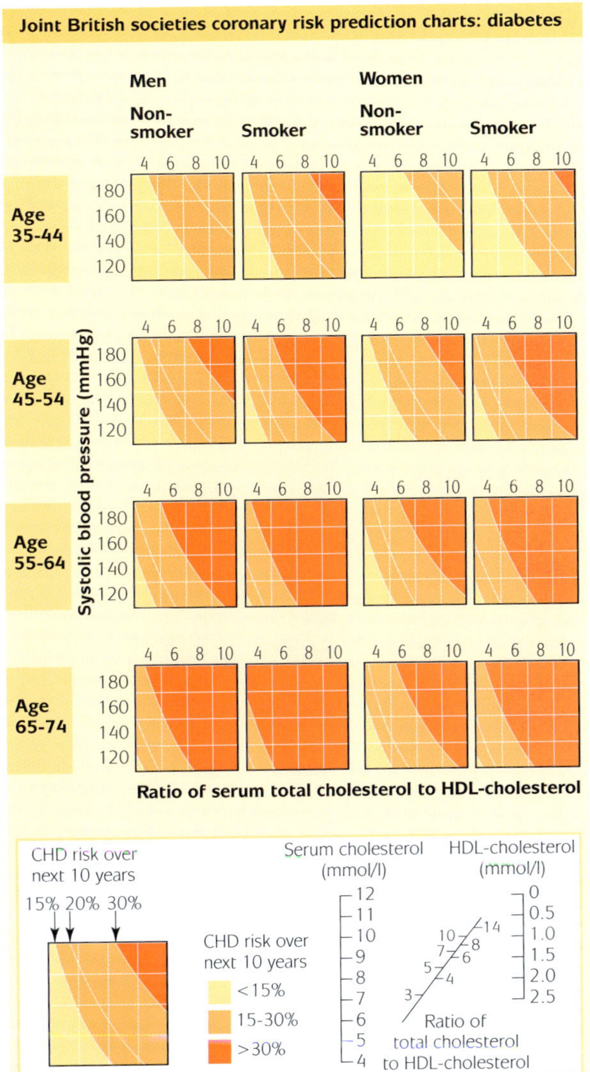

Figure 9. Joint British Societies coronary risk prediction charts for people with diabetes. Reproduced with permission from *BMJ* 2000;**320**:705–708.

LDL-cholesterol goals and cutpoints			
Risk category	**LDL goal**	**LDL level for starting lifestyle changes**	**LDL level for considering drug therapy**
CHD or CHD risk equivalents (10-year risk >20%)	<100 mg/dl	≥100 mg/dl	≥130 mg/dl (100-129 mg/dl: drug optional)**
2 + risk factors (10-year risk ≤20%)	<130 mg/dl	≥130 mg/dl	10-year risk 10-20%: ≥130 mg/dl 10-year risk <10%: ≥160 mg/dl
0-1 risk factor*	<160 mg/dl	≥160 mg/dl	≥190 mg/dl (160-189 mg/dl: LDL-lowering drug optional)

Table 9. LDL-cholesterol goals and cutpoints for therapeutic lifestyle changes and drug therapy in different risk categories. *Almost all people with 0–1 risk factor have a 10-year risk < 10%, thus 10-year risk assessment in people with 0–1 risk factor is not necessary. **Some authorities recommend use of LDL-lowering drugs in this category if an LDL-cholesterol < 100 mg/dl cannot be achieved by therapeutic lifestyle changes. Others prefer use of drugs that primarily modify triglycerides and HDL. Clinical judgement may also call for deferring drug therapy in this subcategory. Reproduced with permission from National Cholesterol Education Program, National Institutes of Health, NIH Publication No. 01-3670, May 2001.

population overestimates coronary and cardiovascular risk in lower-risk Southern European populations.[60,61] As with other epidemiological functions, it also overestimates risk in younger people. Third, the definition of non-fatal endpoints includes new-onset angina, which differs from definitions used in other cohort studies. This makes it difficult to validate the function using data from other studies.

The Systematic Coronary Risk Evaluation (SCORE) project is based on 12 European cohort studies, representing

Estimate of 10-year risk for men

Age	Points
20-34	-9
35-39	-4
40-44	0
45-49	3
50-54	6
55-59	8
60-64	10
65-69	11
70-74	12
75-79	13

	Points				
Total cholesterol	**Age 20-39**	**Age 40-49**	**Age 50-59**	**Age 60-69**	**Age 70-79**
<160	0	0	0	0	0
160-199	4	3	2	1	0
200-239	7	5	3	1	0
240-279	9	6	4	2	1
≥280	11	8	5	3	1

	Points				
	Age 20-39	**Age 40-49**	**Age 50-59**	**Age 60-69**	**Age 70-79**
Non-smoker	0	0	0	0	0
Smoker	8	5	3	1	1

HDL (mg/dl)	Points
≥60	-1
50-59	0
40-49	1
<40	2

Systolic BP (mmHg)	If untreated	If treated
<120	0	0
120-129	0	1
130-139	1	2
140-159	1	2
≥160	2	3

Points total	10-year risk (%)
<0	<1
0	1
1	1
2	1
3	1
4	1
5	2
6	2
7	3
8	4
9	5
10	6
11	8
12	10
13	12
14	16
15	20
16	25
≥17	≥30

Table 10. Ten-year risk assessment for men. Reproduced with permission from National Cholesterol Education Program, National Institutes of Health, NIH Publication No. 01-3670, May 2001.

Estimate of 10-year risk for women

Age	Points
20-34	-7
35-39	-3
40-44	0
45-49	3
50-54	6
55-59	8
60-64	10
65-69	12
70-74	14
75-79	16

Total cholesterol	Points				
	Age 20-39	Age 40-49	Age 50-59	Age 60-69	Age 70-79
<160	0	0	0	0	0
160-199	4	3	2	1	1
200-239	8	6	4	2	1
240-279	11	8	5	3	2
≥280	13	10	7	4	2

	Points				
	Age 20-39	Age 40-49	Age 50-59	Age 60-69	Age 70-79
Non-smoker	0	0	0	0	0
Smoker	9	7	4	2	1

HDL (mg/dl)	Points
≥60	-1
50-59	0
40-49	1
<40	2

Systolic BP (mmHg)	If untreated	If treated
<120	0	0
120-129	1	3
130-139	2	4
140-159	3	5
≥160	4	6

Points total	10-year risk (%)
<9	<1
9	1
10	1
11	1
12	1
13	2
14	2
15	3
16	4
17	5
18	6
19	8
20	11
21	14
22	17
23	22
24	27
≥25	≥30

Table 11. 10-year risk assessment for women. Reproduced with permission from National Cholesterol Education Program, National Institutes of Health, NIH Publication No. 01-3670, May 2001.

a wide range of cardiovascular mortality rates. In round numbers, the SCORE risk prediction system is based on over 200,000 people, 3 million person years of observation and over 7000 fatal cardiovascular events.[54,62] The main features of the SCORE risk prediction system are:

1. The prediction is based on total cardiovascular deaths rather than the combination of non-fatal and fatal events. Non-CHD cardiovascular mortality is especially important because it represents a greater proportion of all cardiovascular risk in European regions with low rates of CHD. An absolute fatal CVD risk greater than 5% from SCORE is equivalent to a CHD event risk greater than 20% based on the Framingham function.
2. A SCORE risk function has been calculated for high- and low-risk European regions. The cohorts from Denmark, Finland and Norway were used to develop the high-risk European region model, and the cohorts from Belgium, Italy and Spain were used to develop the low-risk European region model.
3. The risk in middle-aged subjects, in whom risk changes more rapidly, is provided in more detail.
4. The risk is displayed in each cell as a percentage rather than a broad risk category.
5. The cardiovascular risk is calculated in two ways: one based on total cholesterol and the other on the cholesterol:HDL-cholesterol ratio.

There are several advantages of the SCORE function. First, the function is based on a very large and representative European dataset with hard, reproducible cardiovascular endpoints. Second, fatal CHD and stroke risk can be derived separately. Third, the development of European high- and low-risk region charts improves the applicability of this scoring system across Europe (Figures 10 and 11). Importantly, the risk SCORE function can be customized to any European country based on national mortality data. Therefore, it is possible to produce a risk score chart for each country.

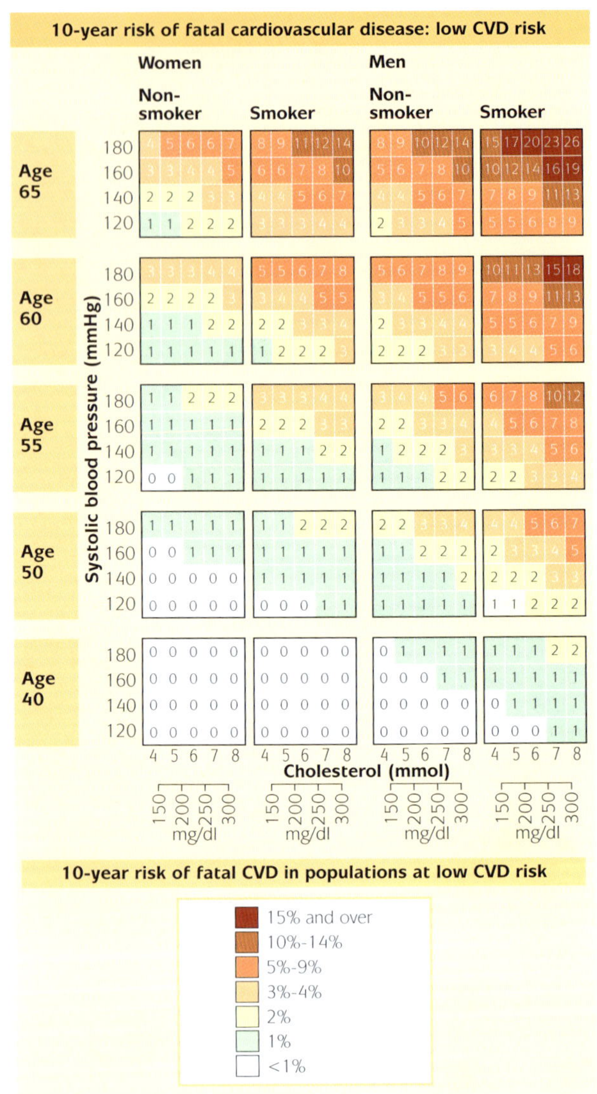

Figure 10. Heart Score chart for predicting 10-year risk of fatal cardiovascular disease in people with a low CVD risk. Reproduced with permission from Conroy RM *et al. Eur Heart J* 2003;**24**:987–1003.

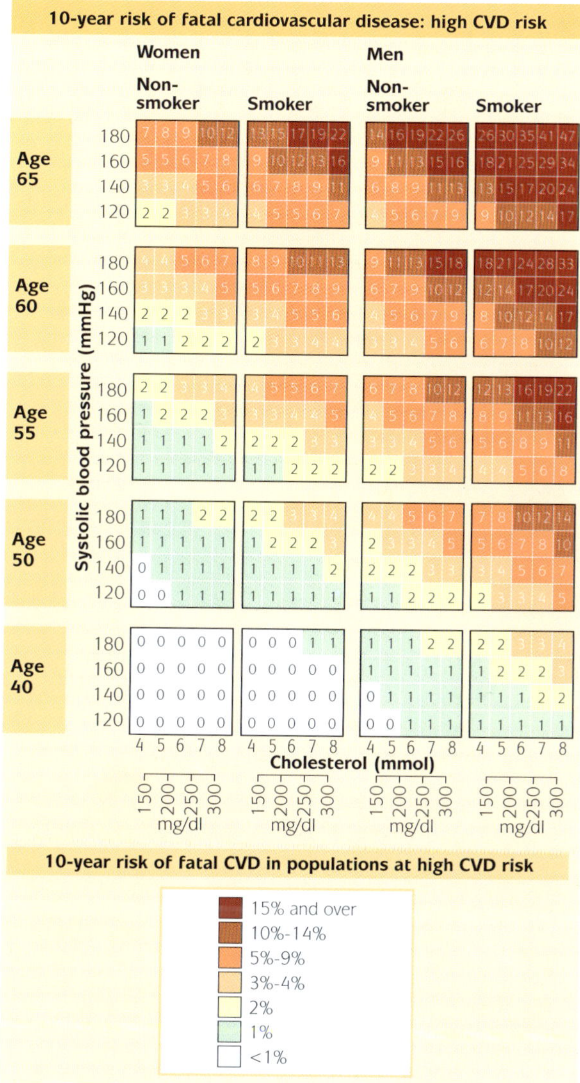

Figure 11. Heart Score chart for predicting 10-year risk of fatal cardiovascular disease in people with a high CVD risk. Reproduced with permission from Conroy RM *et al. Eur Heart J* 2003;**24**:987–1003.

The Heart Score charts have several functions:

- An individual's risk of dying of CVD over the next 10 years can be read from the chart without any calculations.
- The chart illustrates the effect of lifetime risk by showing the increasing risk as age increases.
- Relative risk can be estimated by comparing the risk in one cell with any other cell in the same age group.
- The chart gives some indication of the effect of changing from one risk category to another.

A fatal CVD risk greater than 5% based on Heart Score is considered to be sufficiently high to justify intensive lifestyle interventions and, where appropriate, the use of drug therapies.

Relative risk

Relative risk is the ratio of absolute CHD risk for an individual with one or more risk factors to that of an individual at a reference level of risk. Two different ways of defining the reference level of risk have been used. The first is the absolute risk for a person at low risk (i.e. a person of the same age and sex, but without any major risk factors), and the other is the absolute risk for a person of the same age and sex with average risk in the population. Relative risk informs an individual of their risk in relation to their peers, and is particularly valuable in younger people who are always at low absolute risk.

Lifetime risk

Although young people are always at lower absolute risk than older people, absolute risk will increase as age increases. All the risk charts can be used to estimate lifetime risk by following the horizontal line of boxes upwards to illustrate the effect of risk factor exposure with increasing age if risk factors remain constant or, indeed, if they increase further as age increases. In general, absolute risk will rise even higher than indicated by the charts, since risk factor levels will also tend to increase with age.

Prevention and treatment goals in Europe, and the UK and USA

The lifestyle, risk factor and therapeutic goals in Europe, the UK and the USA for patients with symptomatic atherosclerotic disease and apparently healthy individuals at high multifactorial risk of developing CVD are summarized in Appendix 3.

European guidelines

The European Societies of Cardiology, Atherosclerosis and Hypertension published recommendations on the prevention of CHD in clinical practice in 1994, which were updated by 6 Societies in 1998 and most recently by 8 Societies in 2003.[52-54]

Lifestyle modifications

The specific goals for patients with symptomatic atherosclerotic disease and individuals at high risk of developing CVD are listed in Table12.

Other cardiovascular risk factors

Weight and body shape

The BMI should be maintained at less than 25 kg/m^2. Waist circumference should be less than or equal to 94 cm in men, and less than 80 cm in women.

Blood pressure

The blood pressure goal is consistently below 140/90 mmHg. In diabetic patients, a lower goal of less than 130/80 mmHg is desirable, especially in the presence of nephropathy.

Lifestyle modification goals
• Stop smoking • Make healthy food choices • Increase physical activity

Table 12. Lifestyle modification goals for patients with symptomatic atherosclerotic disease and individuals at high risk of developing CVD.

Blood lipids

The general blood cholesterol goals are:

(i) Total cholesterol consistently below 5.0 mmol/l (190 mg/dl) and

(ii) LDL-cholesterol below 3.0 mmol/l (115 mg/dl).

Concentrations of HDL-cholesterol and triglycerides are not used as goals of therapy.

In patients with established atherosclerotic disease, individuals at high absolute risk of CVD (CVD Heart Score > 5% over 10 years) and those with diabetes mellitus, a lower total cholesterol goal of less than 4.5 mmol/l (175 mg/dl) and an LDL-cholesterol goal of less than 2.5 mmol/l (100 mg/dl) are appropriate if this can be achieved with lipid-lowering drugs for which efficacy and safety have been demonstrated in randomized controlled trials.

Blood glucose

The goals for adequate glucose control in diabetes are shown in Table13.

Prophylactic drug therapies

The following cardioprotective drug classes should be considered in the prevention of CVD.

In patients with established CVD:

- Aspirin or other platelet-modifying drugs in virtually all patients

Goals for glucose control in diabetes
Type 1 diabetes mellitus
1. Fasting blood glucose 5.1–6.5 mmol/l (91–120 mg/dl)
2. Postprandial (peak) glucose 7.6–9.0 mmol/l (136–160 mg/dl)
3. HbA1c 6.0–7.5%
4. Avoidance of serious hypoglycaemias
Type 2 diabetes mellitus
1. Fasting/preprandial (venous plasma) glucose less than 6.0 mmol/l (110 mg/dl), or 4.0–5.0 mmol/l (70–90 mg/dl) for self-monitored blood glucose
2. Postprandial blood glucose 4.0–7.5 mmol/l (70–135 mg/dl)
3. HbA1c less than 6.1%

Table 13. Goals for adequate glucose control in diabetes.

- Beta-blockers in patients following acute MI or with ischaemic cardiomyopathies
- Angiotensin-converting enzyme (ACE) inhibitors in patients with symptoms or signs of heart failure, or left ventricular systolic dysfunction due to CHD and/or arterial hypertension.
- Anticoagulants in patients at increased risk of thromboembolic events because of CHD.

In asymptomatic individuals at high absolute risk of CVD:

- Low-dose aspirin in treated hypertension patients when blood pressure is well controlled, and in men at particularly high risk.

Screening of close relatives

Close relatives of patients with premature CHD (men < 55 years and women < 65 years) and people who belong to families with familial hypercholesterolaemia, or other inherited dyslipidaemias, should be screened for cardiovascular risk factors as they are at increased risk of developing CVD.

UK guidelines

The Joint British Societies (British Cardiac Society, British Hyperlipidaemia Association, British Hypertension Society and the British Diabetes Association) published recommendations on the prevention of CHD in clinical practice in 1998,[55,56] and the British Hypertension Society revised their guidelines in 1999.[63,64] The Joint British recommendations set common lifestyle and risk factor targets for patients with established atherosclerotic disease, and apparently healthy individuals at high absolute risk (Framingham CHD risk > 20% over 10 years) of developing CHD.

Lifestyle, BMI and cholesterol targets for prevention of CHD are the same as those of the Joint European Societies. The only difference is the blood pressure goal, which is less than 140/85 mmHg in the UK. The British recommendations for cardioprotective drug therapies are the same as the European ones.

USA guidelines

In the USA, guidelines for blood pressure and cholesterol are developed by the National High Blood Pressure Education Program (Joint National Committee on Prevention, Detection, Evaluation, and Treatment of High Blood Pressure)[65] and the National Cholesterol Education Program (Expert Panel on Detection, Evaluation, and Treatment of High Blood Cholesterol in Adults).[59] The American Diabetes Association (Expert Committee on the Diagnosis and Classification of Diabetes Mellitus) makes clinical practice recommendations for diabetes.[37,38]

Joint National Committee on Prevention, Detection, Evaluation, and Treatment of High Blood Pressure

The 7th report of the Joint National Committee on Prevention, Detection, Evaluation, and Treatment of High Blood Pressure (JNC VII) recommends treatment of blood pressure based on blood pressure levels alone, irrespective of the context of cardiovascular risk.[65] Calculation of absolute multifactorial risk as a guide to blood pressure management is not recommended.

Hypertension is defined as:

- Stage 1: SBP 140–159 mmHg or DBP 90–99 mmHg; and
- Stage 2: SBP greater than 160 mmHg or DBP greater than 100 mmHg.

The blood pressure goal is less than 140/90 mmHg, or less than 130/80 mmHg in patients with hypertension who also have either diabetes or renal disease.

Expert Panel on Detection, Evaluation, and Treatment of High Blood Cholesterol in Adults

In contrast to the JNC VII, the ATP III recommends treatment of lipids in the context of multifactorial risk.[59] The ATP III classification of LDL, total cholesterol and HDL-cholesterol is presented in Table14. LDL goals are:

1. Less than 2.6 mmol/l (100 mg/dl) for patients with CHD and CHD risk equivalents. CHD risk equivalents comprise:
    - Other clinical forms of atherosclerotic disease
    - Diabetes
    - Multiple risk factors that confer a Framingham 10-year risk for CHD over 20%.
2. Less than 3.4 mmol/l (130 mg/dl) for patients with multiple (two or more) risk factors, but whose Framingham 10-year CHD risk is less than 20%.
3. Less than 4.2 mmol/l (160 mg/dl) for patients with no more than one risk factor.

Classification of cholesterol levels	
LDL-cholesterol (mg/dl)	
<100	Optimal
100 – 129	Near optimal/above optimal
130 – 159	Borderline high
160 – 189	High
≥ 190	Very high
Total cholesterol (mg/dl)	
< 200	Desirable
200 – 239	Borderline high
≥ 240	High
HDL-cholesterol (mg/dl)	
< 40	Low
≥ 60	High

Table 14. ATP III Classification of LDL-cholesterol levels and total and HDL-cholesterol levels. Reproduced with permission from National Cholesterol Education Program, National Institutes of Health, NIH Publication No. 01-3670, May 2001.

Expert Committee on the Diagnosis and Classification of Diabetes Mellitus

The Expert Committee on the Diagnosis and Classification of Diabetes Mellitus defines diagnosis and treatment criteria for diabetes but does not define goals for other cardiovascular risk factors in the context of diabetes.

The blood pressure and lipid goals for diabetes are defined by other Expert Committees as described above.

Lifestyle, risk factor and therapeutic management

Smoking cessation

Behaviour interventions

Physicians should advise all high risk patients to stop smoking completely.[66,67] The momentum for smoking cessation is particularly strong at the time of diagnosing CVD, or when an apparently healthy individual is found to be at high risk of developing CVD. At both hospital clinics and primary care practices, nurses represent an important resource in individual counselling on smoking cessation. There is a strong dose-response relationship between the intensity of tobacco dependence counselling and its effectiveness. Nicotine replacement therapies can initially be helpful for some patients, in particular those who are heavily addicted to nicotine (*see* next section). Support by the spouse/partner and family is also important in smoking cessation. This is because getting other smoking family members to quit tobacco will make it easier for the patient to stop.

Therapeutic interventions

Nicotine replacement therapies are available in the form of nicotine gum, inhaler, nasal spray and patches (*see* Appendix 1).[68] More recently, sustained-release bupropion hydrochloride has been shown to help patients quit smoking. To begin with, nicotine replacement therapy should be prescribed in the absence of contra-indications. Nicotine chewing gum and transdermal nicotine patches can be helpful in the initial weeks or months of smoking cessation. The use of nicotine patches is reported to be safe and without adverse effects in coronary patients. Caution, however, is still required and patients should not smoke while using nicotine replacement therapy.

Dietary intervention

The goal of dietary intervention is to consume a diet associated with the lowest risk of atherosclerotic CVD.

Professional advice

All patients with CVD and high-risk individuals should receive professional advice on food and food choices that make up a diet associated with the lowest risk of atherosclerotic disease. Physicians should emphasize the importance of diet in relation to weight reduction, lowering blood pressure and blood cholesterol, in the control of blood glucose in diabetic patients, and in reducing the propensity to thrombosis. The role of the family is particularly important in this context as the person primarily responsible for buying and preparing food must be informed of the need for healthy food choices and how these can be practically achieved. The relevance of physical activity in helping weight control, and favourably modifying other risk factors, should be explained.

General dietary recommendations

A healthy diet is characterized as one that is low in saturated and *trans* fatty acids and low in dietary cholesterol. The total fat intake should account for no more than 30% of energy intake, and intake of saturated fats should not exceed one-third of total fat intake. Dietary cholesterol intake should be less than 300 mg/day (Table15). Saturated fat can be partly replaced by complex carbohydrates, and partly by monounsaturated and polyunsaturated fats from vegetables and fish. The consumption of the following foods should be encouraged: fruit and vegetables, whole-grain cereals and bread, low-fat diary products, fish and lean meat.

Moderation in the use of alcohol is advised and further restriction may be necessary in those who are overweight (to reduce calories), in particular in hypertensive patients. The intake of salt (sodium chloride) should also be reduced to less than 5 g/day in hypertensive patients.

Table16 give examples of food choices for a healthy lipid-lowering diet. Foods have been grouped into three broad categories: "recommended foods", "foods for use in moderation" and "foods for only exceptional use". General recommendations for food choices with low cardiovascular risk are given in Table 17.

Population goals for nutrients and foods	
Nutrient or food	**Limits for population**
Saturated (and trans) fatty acids (%E)	<10
Polyunsaturated fatty acids (%E)	3-7
Dietary fibre (g/day)	27-40
Fruits and vegetables (g/day)	>400
Legumes, nuts, seeds (g/day)	>30
Cholesterol (mg/day)	<300
Fish (g/d)	>20
Salt (g/d)	<6

Table 15. Population goals for nutrients and foods. Reproduced with permission from Wood D *et al. Eur Heart J* 1998;**19**:1434–1503.

Nutroceuticals

Nutroceuticals are used as dietary supplements. Phytosterols are a group of compounds present in various plants and plant products such as some vegetables and fruits. One of the phytosterols, sitostanol, is now widely available. Phytosterols reduce total cholesterol by 10% and LDL-cholesterol by 13%, and can therefore be helpful as part of a cholesterol-lowering diet. There is currently no clinical trial evidence that dietary supplementation with vitamins or other nutrients is beneficial.

Physical activity

All patients with CHD and high-risk individuals should be professionally encouraged to increase their physical activity safely to the level associated with the lowest risk of CVD. For the healthy population, the goal is to be physically active for 30–45 minutes four to five times weekly. For patients with established CVD, an appropriate exercise prescription is required based on a full clinical assessment including the results, where appropriate, of an exercise tolerance test.

Food choices for a healthy lipid-lowering diet			
	Recommended foods	**Foods used in moderation**	**Foods only for exceptional use**
Cereals	Wholegrain bread, wholegrain breakfast cereals, porridge, cereals, whole grain pasta and rice, crispbread, matzo.	White pasta and rice.	Croissant, brioche.
Dairy products	Skimmed milk, very low-fat cheeses, eg cottage cheese, fat-free fromage frais or quark, fat-free yoghurt, egg white, egg substitutes.	Semi-skimmed milk, fat-reduced and lower fat cheeses eg camembert, edam, feta, ricotta, low-fat yoghurt. Two whole eggs per week.	Whole milk, condensed milk, cream, imitation milk, full-fat cheeses eg brie, gouda, full-fat yoghurt.
Soups	Consommes, vegetable soups.		Thickened soups, cream soups.
Fish	All white and oily fish (grilled, poached, smoked). Avoid skin (eg on sardines or whitebait).	Fish fried in suitable oils.	Roe, fish fried in unknown or unsuitable oils or fats.
Shellfish	Oysters, scallops.	Mussels, lobster, scampi, prawns, shrimps, calamari.	
Meat	Turkey, chicken, veal, game, rabbit, spring lamb. Very lean beef, ham, bacon, lamb (once or twice a week). Veal or chicken sausage. Liver twice a month	Duck, goose, all visibly fatty meats, usual sausages, salamis, meat pies, pates, poultry skin.	
Fats	Polyunsaturated oils eg sunflower, corn, walnut, safflower. Monosaturated oils, (olive oil, rape-seed oil). Soft (unhydrogenated) margarines rich in monounsaturated or polyunsaturated oils, low-fat spreads.		Butter, suet, lard, dripping, palm oil, hard margerines, hydrogenated fats.

Table 16. Food choices for a healthy lipid-lowering diet. Reproduced with permission from Wood D *et al. Eur Heart J* 1998;**19**:1434–1503.

Food choices for a healthy lipid-lowering diet (continued)

	Recommended foods	Foods used in moderation	Foods only for exceptional use
Fruit and vegetables	All fresh and frozen vegetables, emphasis on legumes: beans; dried beans, lentils, chick peas, sweetcorn, boiled or jacket potatoes, all fresh or dried fruit, tinned fruit (unsweetened).	Roast or chipped potatoes cooked in permitted oils.	Roast or chipped potatoes, vegetables or rice fried in unknown or unsuitable oils or fats, potato crisps, oven chips, salted tinned vegetables.
Desserts	Sorbet, jellies, puddings based on skimmed milk, fruit salad, meringue.		Ice cream, puddings, dumplings, sauces based on cream or butter.
Baked foods		Pastry, biscuits prepared with unsaturated margarine or oils.	Commercial pastry, bicuits, commercial pies, snacks and puddings.
Confectionery	Turkish delight, nougat, boiled sweets.	Marzipan, halva.	Chocolate, toffees, fudge, coconut bars, butterscotch.
Nuts	Walnuts, almonds, chestnuts.	Brazils, cashews, peanuts, pistachios.	Coconut, salted nuts.
Beverages	Tea, filter or instant coffee, water, calorie-free soft drinks.	Alcohol, low-fat chocolate drinks.	Chocolate drinks, Irish coffee, full-fat malted drinks, boiled coffee, ordinary soft drinks.
Dressings, flavourings	Pepper, mustard, herbs, spices.	Low-fat salad dressings.	Added salt, salad dressings, salad cream, mayonnaise

1. **"Recommended foods"** are generally low in fat and/or high in fibre. These should be used regularly as part of the diet. The exception is vegetable oils and nuts which are recommended because of their favourable fatty acid composition but, because of their high energy content, should be used in moderation.
2. **"Foods for use in moderation"** contain unsaturated fats or smaller quantities of saturated fats. As the diet should be low in fat, these foods should be used in moderation.
3. **"Foods only for exceptional use"** contain large proportions of saturated or hydrogenated fats and/or cholesterol, or sugar and therefore should be avoided wherever possible.

health status helps in weight reduction and in the maintenance of reduced body weight. A realistic goal for weight reduction is 0.5–1 kg per week until the weight goal is achieved.

Therapeutic interventions

The therapeutic management of obesity includes drugs that reduce food intake, increase energy expenditure and affect nutrient partitioning or metabolism (*see* Appendix 1). Sibutramine, a serotonin-norepinephrine re-uptake inhibitor, decreases food intake, and orlistat, an intestinal lipase inhibitor decreases fat absorption. Clinical trials of *d*-fenfluramine, sibutramine and orlistat have shown that these agents increase body weight loss by an average of 2–4 kg when compared with placebo. More interestingly, the number of patients who succeeded in obtaining and maintaining a reduction of more than 10% of initial body weight has been increased by two to three more times. Sibutramine is recommended for patients with a BMI greater or equal to 30 kg/m^2 without concomitant risk factors, and patients with a BMI greater or equal to 27 kg/m^2 with concomitant risk factors. Sibutramine should be used with caution in patients with a history of hypertension, and should not be used in those with uncontrolled hypertension and concomitant CVD.[73]

Blood pressure

Lifestyle interventions

Several lifestyle interventions are known to have a blood pressure lowering effect (Table19).

A low-salt diet can lower blood pressure and prevent the increase of blood pressure with age. A diet low in dairy produce and high in fruit and vegetables will reduce blood pressure.

These lifestyle modifications can also decrease the number and doses of antihypertensive drugs to control blood pressure.

Therapeutic interventions

Large-scale clinical trials have demonstrated that lowering blood pressure by drugs reduces cardiovascular morbidity

Lifestyle interventions known to have a blood pressure lowering effect
• Weight reduction in overweight individuals • Reduction in the use of sodium chloride to less than 5 g/day • Increasing the intake of potassium from fresh fruit and vegetables • Restriction of alcohol consumption to: – No more than 10–30 g/day ethanol in men (one to three standard measures of spirits, one to three glasses of wine, or one to three bottles of beer) – 10–20 g/day ethanol in women (one to two drinks per day) • Regular physical activity in sedentary individuals

Table 19. Lifestyle interventions that reduce blood pressure.

and mortality, and this benefit extends to the very elderly (up to 80 years of age).

Following the development of CVD, blood pressure elevation is still associated with an increased risk of further non-fatal and fatal cardiovascular events. Several classes of antihypertensive agents (beta-blockers, ACE inhibitors and calcium-channel blockers – not of the dihydropyridine class) have provided cardioprotection to patients following MI. The benefits of antihypertensive drug treatment have also been shown in post-stroke patients.

Five classes of antihypertensive therapies have been shown to reduce cardiovascular morbidity and mortality in the healthy population (Table 20). These are recommended as first-line choice for antihypertensive treatment.

In all trials, blood pressure control has frequently been achieved by the combination of two or even three drugs. Combinations with proven efficacy and tolerability are given in Table 21.

- Some anti-hypertensive drug classes have specific clinical indications. In patients with heart failure due to coronary artery disease, diuretics, ACE inhibitors and

Antihypertensive drugs that reduce cardiovascular morbidity and moratily in healthy populations
• Diuretics • Beta-blockers • ACE inhibitors • Calcium-channel blockers • Angiotensin II antagonists

Table 20. Antihypertensive therapies shown to reduce cardiovascular morbidity and mortality in the healthy population.

Antihypertensive drug combinations
• A diuretic with a beta-blocker, or an ACE inhibitor or an angiotensin II antagonist
• A beta-blocker with a long-acting dihydropyridine calcium antagonist or an alpha-blocker
• An ACE inhibitor with a calcium-channel blocker

Table 21. Antihypertensive drug combinations with proven efficacy and tolerability.

beta-blockers are preferred. The latter agents are only used after the patient's condition is stabilized, and at very low doses with slow up-titration under careful supervision.

- In patients with asymptomatic left ventricular dysfunction, ACE inhibitors and beta-blockers are appropriate. Following MI, beta-blockers and ACE inhibitors provide cardiovascular protection.
- In patients with stable angina pectoris beta-blockers or calcium-channel blockers should be used to control symptoms as well as reaching the blood pressure goal. ACE inhibitors are also appropriate for blood pressure reduction.

- ACE inhibitors, and also calcium-channel blockers are indicated in diabetic individuals as well as in patients with a high cardiovascular risk profile:
  - Angiotensin-II antagonists in patients with Type 2 diabetic nephropathy and ACE inhibitors in non-diabetic nephropathy
  - ACE inhibitors and diuretics in patients with a history of cerebrovascular disease
  - Diuretics and calcium antagonists in black patients (with low priority for ACE inhibitors and angiotensin-II antagonists).

When to start anti-hypertensive therapy?

In patients with acute CVD the initiation of blood pressure lowering therapy depends on the patients overall cardiovascular status. In acute myocardial infarction a beta-blocker and an ACE inhibitor may both be started during the hospital admission if there are no contraindications. Anti-hypertensive treatments may also be started early in patients with other forms of acute atherosclerotic disease. In the recovery phase systematic blood pressure monitoring is required and, if appropriate, anti-hypertensive drug therapy started or up-titrated to ensure all patients with established CVD have a blood pressure level consistently below 140/90 mm Hg (or lower in selected patient groups).

In apparently healthy high-risk individuals the initiation of blood pressure lowering therapy depends on both the blood pressure level and the absolute CVD risk (Figure 12).

The goal is effective blood pressure reduction to target levels as defined in International and National Guidelines (Appendix 3) using all appropriate drugs and drug combinations required.

Lipids

Lifestyle interventions

All patients with CVD and high-risk individuals should follow the dietary recommendations already described.

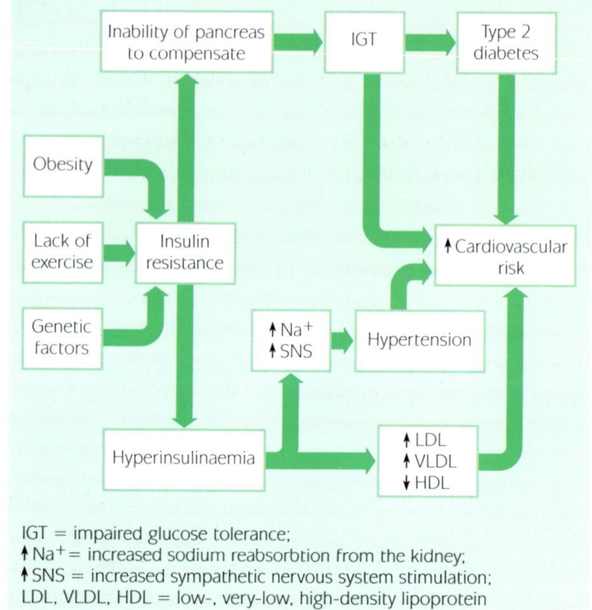

Figure 12. The metabolic syndrome hypothesis. This relates the common combination of cardiovascular risk factors to insulin resistance. Reproduced with permission from Barnett AH, O'Gara G. *In Clinical Practice: Diabetes and the Heart*. London: Churchill Livingstone, 2003.

Therapeutic interventions

Large-scale clinical trials have demonstrated that cholesterol-lowering, principally by inhibitors of HMG-CoA reductase (statins), reduces cardiovascular morbidity and mortality in both patients with established CVD and those at high risk of developing CVD.

Secondary causes of dyslipidaemia should always be excluded before beginning treatment. These include alcohol abuse, diabetes, hypothyroidism, liver and kidney diseases, and concomitant use of several drugs. Some patients with particularly abnormal lipid levels could have genetic diseases such as familial hypercholesterolaemia and should, wherever possible, be referred for specialist evaluation. In familial hypercholesterolaemia, total cholesterol is usually over 8.0 mmol/l (320 mg/dl) with an LDL-cholesterol level higher than 6.0 mmol/l (240 mg/dl) and often a family history of premature CHD. Elevated triglycerides over 5.0 mmol/l (450 mg/dl) may also require specialist opinion.

Lipid-lowering drugs

The current armamentarium of lipid-lowering drugs can be divided into five classes (Table 22). The first four classes of drugs, but not all drugs within each class, have been shown in clinical trials to reduce CHD, and at least one drug class has been shown to reduce CVD.

Statins

The most convincing evidence from clinical trials has been obtained with the most potent lipid-lowering drugs – the statins. These agents also have a good safety record, and are the easiest to use. Statin drugs are currently used first line for lowering LDL-cholesterol. They vary in the degree to which they reduce LDL and in other properties such as antithrombotic and anti-inflammatory effects.

Clinical practice should be based on evidence from major trials with hard clinical endpoints and safety data. The statins used in such trials now published are pravastatin, simvastatin, lovastatin, atorvastatin and, most recently, fluvastatin. The newest available statin is rosuvastatin and this is currently

Lipid-lowering drugs
• Inhibitors of HMG-CoA reductase (statins)
• Fibrates
• Bile-acid sequestrants (anion-exchange resins)
• Nicotinic acid and its derivatives
• Cholesterol-absorption inhibitors

Table 22. Five classes of lipid-lowering drugs.

being evaluated in clinical trials. Although long-term trials have indicated that the statins are quite safe, post-marketing surveillance has shown that cerivastatin, especially when given in conjunction with other drugs such as fibrates, can cause fatal rhabdomyolysis and death. Therefore, preference should be given to those statins for which there is both clinical trial efficacy and safety data.

Fibrates

Fibrates lower triglycerides and increase HDL cholesterol. The evidence from clinical trials to support the use of fibrates is not as good as that supporting the statins, but new clinical trials of fibrates are in progress.

Bile-acid sequestrants and nicotinic acid

Anion-exchange resins and nicotinic acid (niacin) are both useful and safe, but their use is limited by side effects such as constipation and flushing. A new bile acid sequestrant with greater tolerability called colesevelam is being evaluated.

Cholesterol-absorption drugs

A new class of lipid-lowering drugs that inhibits cholesterol absorption from the small intestine (ezetimibe) is now available and is being evaluated in clinical trials.

Drug combinations

Lipid-lowering drugs can be used in combination. For example, the combination of a bile-acid sequestrant and a statin is currently used in practice, and even a triple regimen of a bile-acid sequestrant, a statin and niacin can be useful in some patients. Statins can also be combined with fibrates, but this combination has been associated with myopathy and, although rarely fatal, rhabdomyolysis, and patients must be carefully selected and carefully instructed about warning symptoms (myalgia). The combination of a statin with a cholesterol-absorption inhibitor is being evaluated and could turn out to be valuable.

When to start lipid-lowering therapy?

For patients with an acute MI, a statin should be prescribed in hospital, together with professional dietary advice. The only disadvantage of this approach is that an accurate estimation of untreated plasma lipids will not be available, given the acute-phase response of plasma lipids to MI. Therefore, it is important to measure fasting lipids about 3 months after the acute event, and to modify treatment to ensure the lipid targets are achieved. It is also necessary to consider whether the patient has a genetically determined dyslipidaemia requiring family investigation.

In apparently healthy high-risk individuals the initiation of lipid lowering therapy depends on the absolute CVD risk (Figure 12).

The goal is effective total and LDL-cholesterol reduction to target levels as defined in International and National Guidelines (Appendix 3).

Glycaemia and diabetes

Lifestyle interventions

In Type 2 diabetes, professional dietary advice, weight and central obesity reduction, and increased physical activity are all required for good glucose control.

The precursor stages of Type 2 diabetes – IGT and impaired fasting glycaemia (IFG) – are already associated with an increased risk of cardiovascular disease (Figure 12). Therefore, if IGT and IFG are diagnosed, in particular in a person who has a family history of Type 2 diabetes, it is prudent to start diet interventions and weight reduction, as well as to increase physical activity, with the aim of improving glucose tolerance. Correction of other cardiovascular risk factors is equally important for such individuals as it is for patients with clinically manifest diabetes.

Therapeutic interventions

The results from clinical trials have shown that good metabolic control in Type 1 and Type 2 diabetes prevents microvascular complications, and that the risk of complications can be reduced by management of blood pressure (Figure 13) and lipids (Figure14). In Type 1 diabetes, glucose control requires insulin therapy and professional dietary advice. If the lifestyle measures mentioned earlier do not sufficiently reduce hyperglycaemia in patients with Type 2 diabetes, then treatment with oral hypoglycaemic drugs (sulphonylurea or biguanide, or their combination) or insulin are required. In overweight or obese patients, metformin is the optimal treatment.

Self-monitoring of blood glucose is essential in the treatment of Type 1 diabetes to improve the safety and quality of treatment, and is a vital safeguard against serious hypoglycaemia (Figure 15). Self-monitoring is also recommended for patients with Type 2 diabetes treated with sulphonylureas or insulin.

Blood pressure and cholesterol also need to be treated in patients with diabetes. For blood pressure, the goal is less than 130/80 mmHg, in particular for those with diabetic nephropathy and proteinuria. ACE inhibitors and angiotensin-II receptor

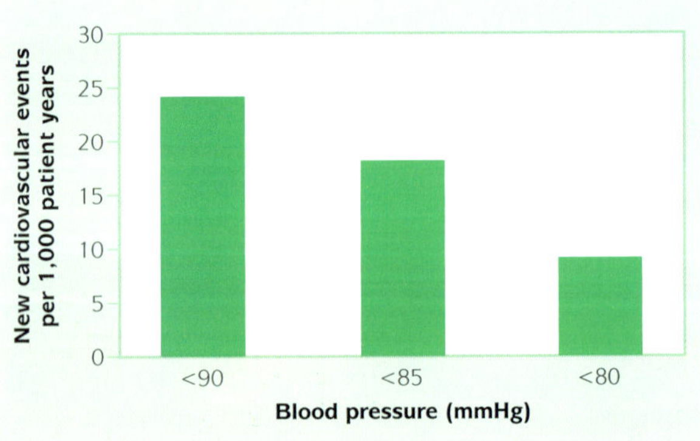

Figure 13. In the Hypertension Optimal Treatment study, cardiovascular endpoint and mortality were halved in patients with Type 2 diabetes randomized to "tight" compared with "least tight" blood pressure control. Source: Hansson L, Zanchetti A, Carruthers SG *et al. Lancet* 1998;**351**:1755–1762.

blockers are particularly effective at preventing progression from micro-albuminuria to overt nephropathy in diabetes, and are the preferred drug classes. The total cholesterol goal for diabetes is less than 4.5 mmol/l (170 mg/dl), and the LDL-cholesterol goal is less than 2.5 mmol/l (100 mg/dl).

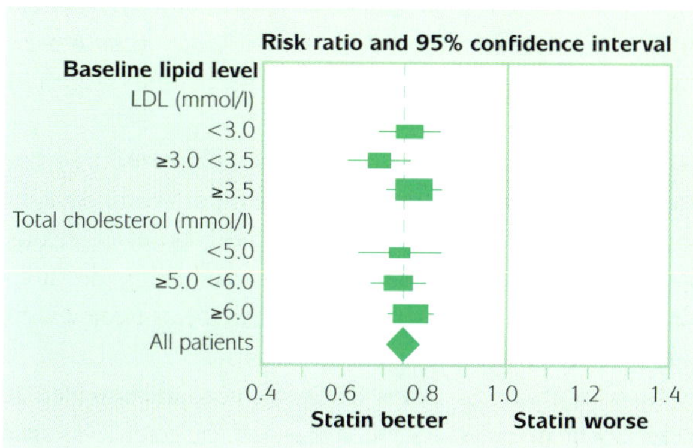

Figure 14. Vascular event by prior lipid levels in the Heart Protection Study. Reproduced from the Heart Protection Study Collaborative Group. *The Lancet* 2002;**360**:7–22. With permission from Elsevier Ltd.

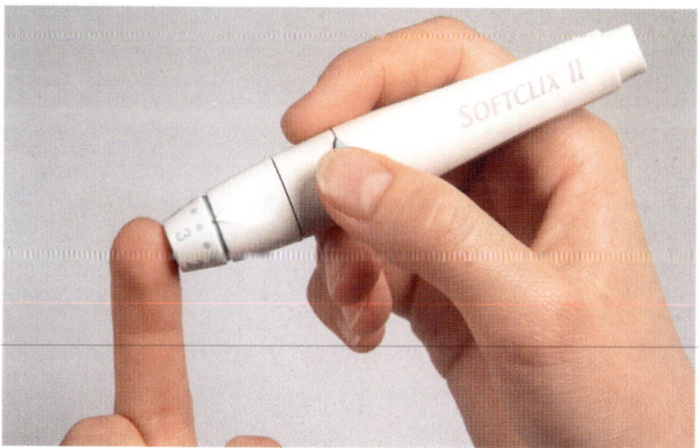

Figure 15. Self-monitoring of blood glucose is essential in the treatment of type 1 diabetes. Reproduced with permission from Professor Pierre-Jean Guillausseau.

Satins currently represent the drug class of choice. The same blood pressure and cholesterol goals are appropriate in patients with the precursors of diabetes.

Prophylactic drug therapies

Antithrombotic drugs

Antiplatelet and anticoagulant medications play an important therapeutic role in the prevention of CVD.[74] Randomized controlled trials have shown the beneficial effect of antiplatelet drugs in the prevention of cardiovascular events. Furthermore, the meta-analysis of clinical trials provides convincing evidence that the administration of antiplatelets following MI significantly reduces all-cause mortality, vascular mortality, non-fatal re-infarction of the myocardium and non-fatal stroke (Figure 16). It is therefore recommended that platelet-modifying drugs should be prescribed in virtually all patients with CHD or other atherosclerotic disease.[75,76]

Aspirin

In trials with aspirin, the most widely tested doses ranged between 75 and 325 mg daily.[77,78] There was no evidence of any greater clinical benefit for doses between 160 and 325 mg daily compared with 75 mg daily. Side effects from aspirin use, principally gastro-intestinal bleeding and peptic ulceration, are lowest in those using 75mg or less daily. Therefore:

- A maintenance dose of 75 mg of aspirin daily is recommended for all patients following MI and those with other clinical manifestations of coronary artery disease such as unstable and stable angina.
- Although there is no long-term (beyond a few years) clinical evidence, it would be both prudent and safe to continue aspirin therapy for life.
- For patients with stroke or transient ischaemic attacks, aspirin at a dose of at least 75 mg daily is recommended and should also be considered for other high-risk patients with peripheral arterial disease.

- In high-risk individuals (e.g. treated hypertensive patients whose blood pressure is well controlled[79] and men at particularly high CHD risk[80]), aspirin at 75 mg daily should be considered.

A recent meta-analysis of aspirin for primary prevention showed that the absolute therapeutic benefits and safety were related to coronary risk. Aspirin treatment for primary prevention was:

- Safe and worthwhile at a coronary risk of at least 15% over 10 years
- Safe but of limited value at a coronary risk of 10% over 10 years,
- Unsafe at a coronary risk of 5% over 10 years.

Therefore, prescribing aspirin for primary prevention of CVD requires formal estimation of coronary or cardiovascular risk.[81]

Other antiplatelet drugs

When aspirin cannot be tolerated, alternative antiplatelet therapies should be considered. The newer antiplatelet drug clopidogrel at a dose of 75 mg daily has been shown to be safe and effective for prevention in those with established CVD.[82] The annual incidence of MI, ischaemic stroke or vascular death is significantly reduced by clopidogrel in the Clopidogrel versus Aspirin in Patients at Risk of Ischaemic Events (CAPRIE) trial (Figure17).[83]

Other antiplatelet drugs such as ticlodipine and dipyridamole are no more effective than aspirin. Ticlodipine has been used alone or in combination with aspirin, but serious adverse effects have limited its use.

Anticoagulants

Anticoagulants are only indicated in selected patients who are at increased risk of thromboembolic events, including those with large anterior MI, left ventricular aneurysm or thrombus, paroxysmal tachyarrhythmias or chronic heart failure, and patients with a history of thromboembolic events.[84,85]

Category of trial	No. of trials with data	No. (%) of vascular events	
		Allocated antiplatelet	Adjusted control
Previous myocardial infarction	12	1345/9984 (13.5)	1708/10,022 (17.0)
Acute myocardial infarction	15	1007/9658 (10.4)	1370/9644 (14.2)
Previous stroke/ transient ischaemic attack	21	2045/11,493 (17.8)	2464/11,527 (21.4)
Acute stroke	7	1670/20,418 (8.2)	1858/20,403 (9.1)
Other high risk	140	1638/20,359 (8.0)	2102/20,543 (10.2)
Subtotal: all except acute stroke	188	6035/51,494 (11.7)	7644/51,736 (14.8)
All trials	**195**	**7705/71,912 (10.7)**	**9502/72,139 (13.2)**

Heterogeneity of odds reductions between:
5 categories of trial: $\chi^2 = 21.4$, df = 4; $P = 0.0003$
Acute stroke v other: $\chi^2 = 18.0$, df = 1; $P = 0.00002$

Figure 16. Proportional effect of antiplatelet therapy on vascular events (myocardial infarction, stroke or vascular death) in five main high-risk categories of patients. For each group of trials, a black square indicates the plot of an event's stratified odds ratio in treatment groups to that in control groups, with a horizontal line representing its 99% confidence interval; the open diamonds denote the meta-analysis results for all trials (95% confidence interval). Reproduced with permission from *BMJ* 2002;**324**:71–86.

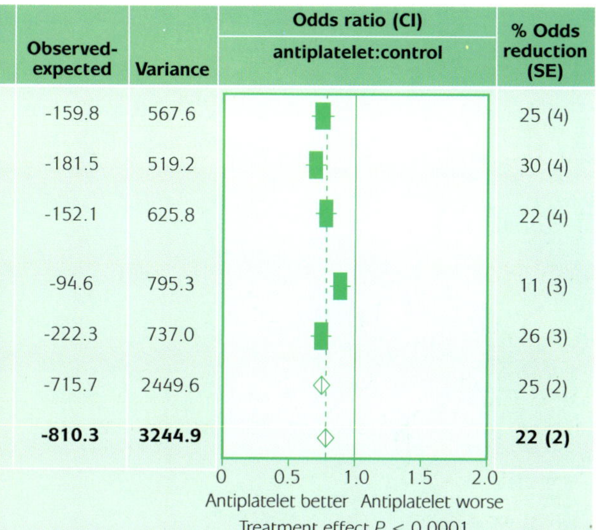

Observed-expected	Variance	Odds ratio (CI) antiplatelet:control	% Odds reduction (SE)
-159.8	567.6		25 (4)
-181.5	519.2		30 (4)
-152.1	625.8		22 (4)
-94.6	795.3		11 (3)
-222.3	737.0		26 (3)
-715.7	2449.6		25 (2)
-810.3	**3244.9**		**22 (2)**

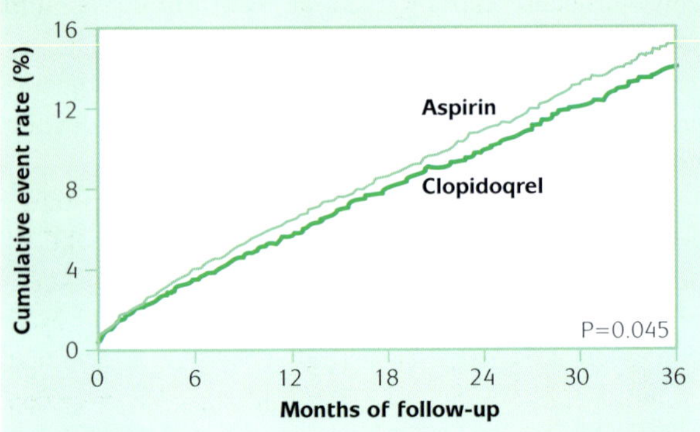

Figure 17. In the CAPRIE trial clopidogrel was associated with a lower incidence of cardiovascular outcome events than aspirin.

Beta-blockers

Beta-blockers are indicated in patients following acute MI.[86-93] In a meta-analysis of beta adrenoceptor antagonists following MI, there was a significant reduction in all-cause mortality, in particular sudden cardiac death, and non-fatal re-infarction (Figure 18). This clinical benefit was greatest in those patients with left ventricular dysfunction, or supraventricular or ventricular tachyarrhythmias.

Therefore, a beta-blocker should be considered in patients with no contraindications following MI, in particular high-risk patients because of mechanical or electrical complications. More recent clinical evidence has shown that beta-blockers can reduce mortality in patients with chronic symptomatic heart failure because of left ventricular systolic dysfunction. This reinforces the need for beta-blockade in coronary patients.

Angiotensin-converting enzyme inhibitors/angiotensin-II receptor blockers

Angiotensin-converting enzyme inhibitors

ACE inhibitors are indicated in patients following acute MI (Table 23). These agents have been shown to significantly reduce all-cause mortality and the risk of progression to persistent heart failure in patients with symptoms or signs of heart failure at the time of acute MI, those with a large MI and in those with left ventricular systolic dysfunction (estimated ejection fraction < 40%).[94-97]

Large long-term clinical trials, including the Cooperative North Scandinavian Enalapril Survival Study (CONSENSUS-I), Survival and Ventricular Enlargement (SAVE), Acute Infarction Ramipril Efficacy (AIRE), Trandolapril Cardiac Evaluation (TRACE) and Study of Left Ventricular Dysfunction (SOLVD), have confirmed that ACE inhibition decreases heart failure, MI and mortality, and that this clinical benefit can be observed within 30 days. The Heart Outcomes Prevention Evaluation (HOPE) trial provides further evidence of the benefits of ACE inhibition in patients with coronary disease and preserved left ventricular function.[98] In this trial, a 22% relative risk reduction of the combined endpoint of death, MI and stroke was obtained using ramipril 10 mg once daily (Figure19). The indication for ACE inhibitors has been extended to all patients with stable coronary disease with the results from the European Trial on Reduction of Cardiac Events with Perindopril (EUROPA) using perindopril at 8 mg daily during the mean follow-up period of 4.2 years (Table 24).[99] The study showed a 20% relative risk reduction of the primary endpoint which was cardiovascular death, myocardial infarction, or cardiac arrest.

Angiotensin-II receptor antagonists

Angiotensin-II receptor antagonists are a newer class of drugs with an antihypertensive effect equivalent to that of an ACE inhibitor, but with better tolerance and no class-specific adverse effects. Clinical trials have shown that these agents are able to significantly reduce cardiovascular morbidity and mortality in high-risk patients with arterial hypertension or diabetes. The results of the Losartan Intervention For Endpoint (LIFE) study show that, compared with atenolol, losartan prevented more cardiovascular morbidity and mortality (Figure 20), as well as all-cause mortality (Figure 21).[100,101]

Trial	Weight (%)	Odds ratio (95% CI)
Boissel 1990	2.9	0.49 (0.25 to 0.93)
Acebutolol pooled	2.9	0.49 (0.25 to 0.93)
Reynolds 1972	0.3	1.03 (0.13 to 8.21)
Ahlmark 1974	0.8	0.58 (0.15 to 1.94)
Wilhelmsson 1974	1.2	0.48 (0.16 to 1.33)
Andersen 1979	4.3	0.96 (0.62 to 1.47)
Alprenolol pooled	6.6	0.83 (0.59 to 1.17)
Wilcox 1980	0.1	1.02 (0.48 to 2.16)
Yusuf 1979	1.5	1.00 (0.01 to 86.25)
Atenolol pooled	1.6	1.02 (0.52 to 1.99)
Basu 1997	0.3	0.62 (0.05 to 5.61)
Carvedilol pooled	0.3	0.62 (0.05 to 5.61)
Rehnqvist 1980	0.7	0.56 (0.11 to 2.53)
Lopez 1993	1.4	1.91 (0.76 to 5.05)
Manger Cats 1983	2.4	0.55 (0.21 to 1.36)
Rehnqvist 1984	4.6	0.73 (0.39 to 1.35)
Salathia 1985	5.4	0.76 (0.49 to 1.18)
LIT Research Group 1987	7.9	0.92 (0.67 to 1.27)
Hjalmarson 1981	0.5	0.62 (0.40 to 0.96)
Metoprolol pooled	23.1	0.80 (0.66 to 0.96)
European infarction study 1984	1.0	1.33 (0.87 to 2.04)
Schwartz 1992 (high risk)	2.4	0.16 (0.02 to 0.79)
Schwartz 1992 (low risk)	3.8	0.53 (0.26 to 1.06)
Taylor 1982	4.6	0.92 (0.61 to 1.41)
Oxprenolol pooled	11.8	0.91 (0.71 to 1.17)
Australian and Swedish study 1983	3.6	0.96 (0.60 to 1.55)
Pindolol pooled	3.6	0.96 (0.60 to 1.55)
Barber 1967	2.9	0.87 (0.51 to 1.50)
Multicentre International study 1975	11.0	0.78 (0.59 to 1.03)
Practolol pooled	13.9	0.80 (0.63 to 1.02)
Kaul 1988	2.4	1.00 (0.12 to 8.31)
Mazur 1984	0.2	0.44 (0.11 to 1.43)
Wilcox 1980	1.5	0.86 (0.40 to 1.84)
Baber 1980	2.3	1.07 (0.59 to 1.93)
Aronow 1997	3.1	0.40 (0.19 to 0.83)
Hansteen 1982	16.0	0.65 (0.37 to 1.15)
BHAT Trial Research Group 1982	1.0	0.72 (0.56 to 0.91)
Propranolol pooled	29.6	0.71 (0.59 to 0.85)
Julian 1982	5.3	0.81 (0.54 to 1.21)
Solalol pooled	5.3	0.81 (0.54 to 1.21)
Roqué 1987	1.0	0.53 (0.17 to 1.54)
Norwegian Multicentre Study Group 1981	12.6	0.60 (0.45 to 0.79)
Timolol pooled	13.6	0.59 (0.46 to 0.77)
Darasz 1995	0.1	3.45 (0.25 to 188.83)
Xamoterol pooled	0.1	3.45 (0.25 to 188.83)
Fixed effects pooled	**100**	**0.77 (0.70 to 0.84)**
Full random effects pooled	**100**	**0.77 (0.69 to 0.85)**

Heterogeneity Q = 39.7, df = 32, $P = 0.16$

Figure 18. Odds ratio (rectangles) of death and pooled odds ratios (diamonds) in long-term trials with beta-blockers (LIT = lopressor intervention; BHAT = beta-blocker heart attack trial). Reprinted with permission from *BMJ* 1999;**318**:1730–1377.

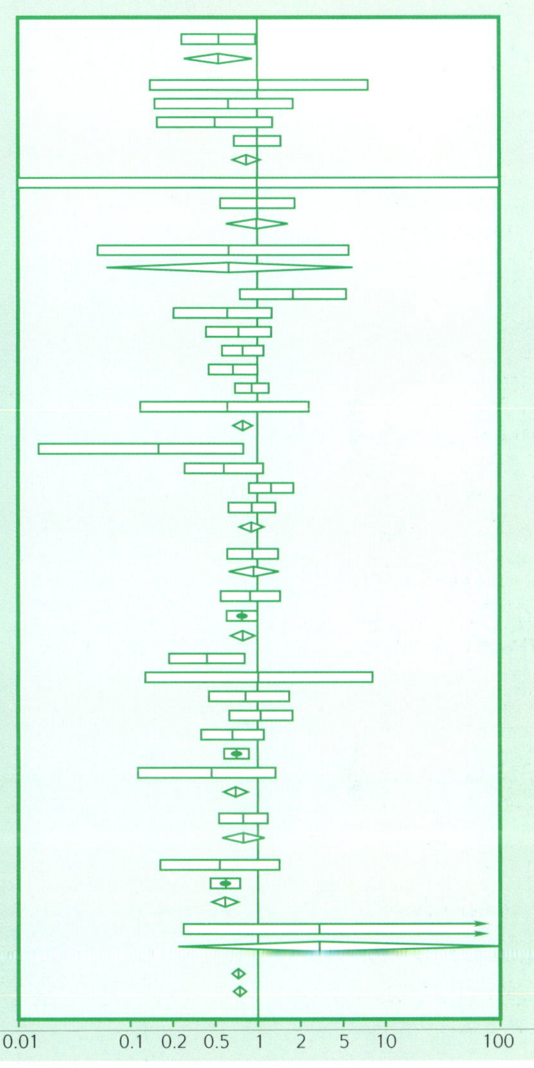
0.01
0.1
0.2
0.5
1
2
5
10
100

Baseline characteristics					
	Sample size		Total mortality		
Study	**ACE**	**Placebo**	**ACE**	**Placebo**	**OR (95% CI)**
Mortarino	10	11	0	0	1.10 (0.02-60.30)
Oldroyd	49	50	8	5	1.69 (0.54-5.36)
Nabel	20	18	0	1	0.29 (0.01-7.44)
Sharpe	50	50	3	2	1.43 (0.27-7.61)
SMILE	772	784	50	65	0.77 (0.52-1.12)
EDI	47	42	1	0	2.74 (0.11-69.15)
ECCE	104	104	2	3	0.71 (0.14-3.67)
CONSENSUS 2	3044	3046	312	286	1.10 (0.93-1.31)
SAVE	1115	1116	228	275	0.79 (0.64-0.96)
AIRE	1004	982	170	222	0.70 (0.56-0.87)
PRACTICAL	150	75	12	12	0.46 (0.20-1.06)
Søgaard	29	29	1	1	1.00 (0.10-10.20)
CATS	149	149	13	10	1.31 (0.57-3.05)
TRACE	876	873	304	369	0.73 (0.60-0.88)
EDEN	239	117	1	0	1.48 (0.06-36.56)
Overall	**7658**	**7446**	**1105**	**1251**	**0.83 (0.71-0.97)**

ACE = angiotensin-converting enzyme inhibitor treated group; CI = confidence interval; OR = random effects odds ratio; Placebo = placebo treated group.

Table 23. Effect of angiotensin-converting enzyme inhibitor on risk of death in patients following myocardial infarction – total mortality results. Reproduced from *J Am Coll Cardiol* 1999;**33**:598–604; copyright 1999. With permission from the American College of Cardiology Foundation.

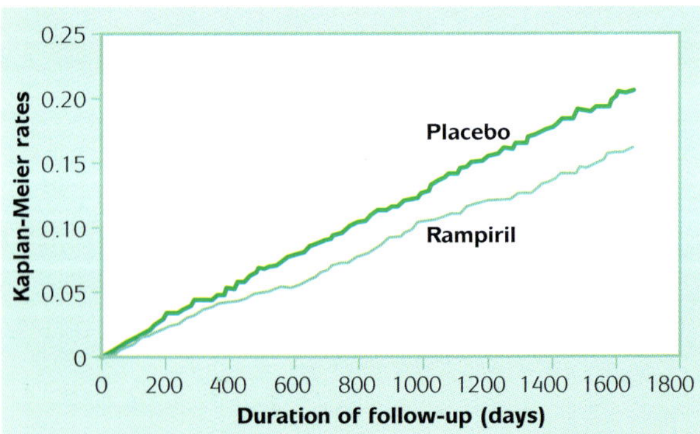

Figure 19. Ramipril significantly reduced the combined primary outcome of MI, stroke or cardiovascular death compared with placebo in the HOPE study of people with diabetes mellitus. Reproduced with permission from *Lancet* 2000;**355**:253–259.

Frequency of primary and selected secondary outcomes				
	Perindopril (n = 6110)	**Placebo (n = 6108)**	**Relative risk reduction (95% CI)**	***p***
Cardiovascular mortality, MI, or cardiac arrest	488 (8.0%)	603 (9-9%)	20% (9 to 29)	0.0003
Cardiovascular mortality	215 (3.5%)	249 (4.1%)	14% (-3 to 28)	0.107
Non-fatal MI	295 (4.8%)	378 (6.2%)	22% (10 to 33)	0.001
Cardiac arrest	6 (0.1%)	11 (0.2%)	46% (-47 to 80)	0.22
Total mortality, non-fatal MI, unstable angina, cardiac arrest	904 (14.8%)	1043 (17.1%)	14% (6 to 21)	0.0009
Total mortality	375 (6.1%)	420 (6.9%)	11% (-2 to 23)	0.1

Table 24. Frequency of primary and selected secondary outcomes (EUROPA trial). Reproduced from *The Lancet* 2003;**362**:782–788. With permission from Elsevier Ltd.

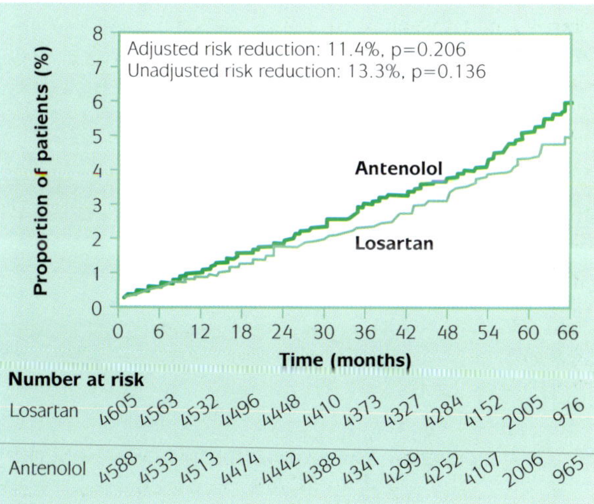

Figure 20. Greater relative risk reduction with losartan compared with atenolol for cardiovascular mortality in the LIFE study. Reproduced with permission from *Lancet* 2002;**359**:995–1003.

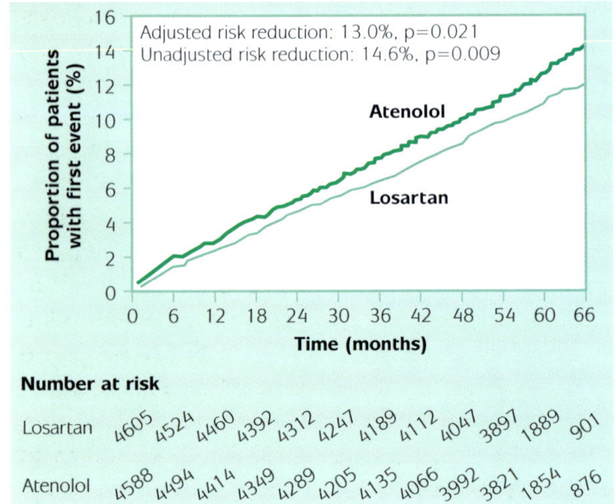

Figure 21. Greater relative risk reduction with losartan compared with atenolol for all-cause mortality in the LIFE study. Reproduced with permission from *Lancet* 2002;**359**:995–1003.

Losartan confers similar reduction in blood pressure as does atenolol, but with better tolerability in patients with hypertension, diabetes and left ventricular hypertrophy. Losartan also significantly reduces cardiovascular outcomes and provides renoprotective effects in patients with Type 2 diabetes and nephropathy in the Reduction of Endpoints in NIDDM with Angiotensin II Antagonist Losartan (RENAAL) study.[102]

Lipid-lowering drugs

Statins

The evidence that cholesterol-lowering is beneficial in patients with coronary disease comes from three landmark clinical trials: Scandinavian Simvastatin Survival Study (4S),[103] Cholesterol and Recurrent Events (CARE)[104] and Long-Term Intervention with Pravastatin in Ischaemic Disease (LIPID).[105] The results from these studies show that simvastatin and pravastatin reduce coronary morbidity and mortality and prolong survival in coronary patients.

In the 4S study, the first of the large-scale clinical trials, simvastatin 20–40 mg daily during 5.4 years reduced coronary and total mortality by 30% and 42%, respectively, in patients with CHD and mean plasma cholesterol concentrations of 6.8 mmol/l. These results were confirmed by another two secondary prevention trials using pravastatin (CARE and LIPID). The CARE study was an intervention trial on patients with CHD and mean plasma cholesterol concentrations of 5.4 mmol/l. After 5 years of treatment, pravastatin 40 mg/daily reduced the incidence of fatal and non-fatal CHD events by 24%. In the LIPID trial, pravastatin 40 mg/daily during 6.1 years mean follow-up period reduced the relative risk of death from CHD by 24%, the overall mortality by 22%, incidence of myocardial infarction by 29% and coronary revascularisation by 20% in patients with a broad range of initial cholesterol levels.

In primary prevention, the results from the West of Scotland Coronary Prevention Study (WOSCOPS)[106] and the Air Force/Texas Coronary Prevention Study (AFCAPS/ TexCAPS)[107] demonstrate similar benefits in high- and low-risk healthy populations with dyslipidaemia. The WOSCOPS trial included patients without CHD and mean plasma cholesterol concentrations of 7.0 mmol/l. After about 5 years of treatment, pravastatin 40 mg/daily reduced the relative risk of major coronary events by 31% and total deaths by 22%. The Air Force/Texas Coronary Atherosclerosis Prevention Study (AFCAPS/ TexCAPS) was carried out on healthy patients with mean plasma cholesterol concentrations of 5.7 mmol/l and below-average HDL-cholesterol levels. After about 5.2 years of treatment, lovastatin 20–40 mg/daily, in addition to a diet low in saturated fat and cholesterol, reduced the incidence of major acute CHD events (fatal or non-fatal MI, unstable angina or sudden cardiac death) by 37% (Figure 22).

The results of a more recent study, the Heart Protection Study, show that lipid-lowering with simvastatin at a daily dose of 40 mg during 5 years safely reduces the risk of major vascular events in a wide range of high-risk individuals with

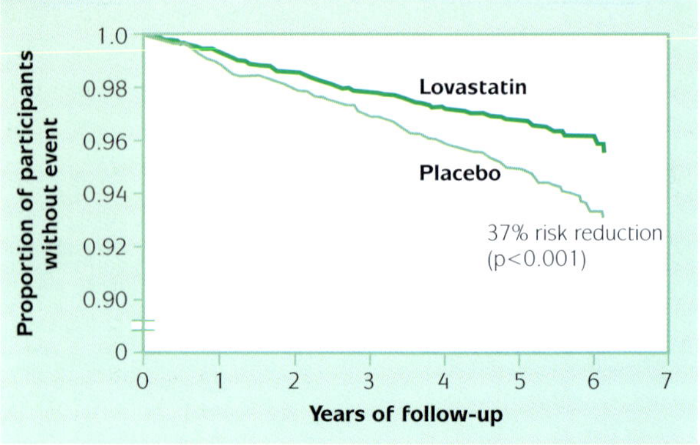

Figure 22. In the AFCAPS/TEXCAPS trial lovastatin reduced the incidence of major acute CHD events during a median of 5.1 years follow up. Reproduced with permission from *JAMA* 1998;**279**:1615–1622.

mean plasma cholesterol concentrations greater than 3.5 mmol/l at baseline.[108] This benefit was also seen in individuals presenting with a low baseline LDL-cholesterol level (< 3 mmol/l). All individuals at high risk or with atherosclerotic disease could therefore potentially benefit from treatment with lipid-lowering drugs, irrespective of their plasma cholesterol concentrations.

The treatment with pravastatin in the CARE study also reduced stroke significantly by 31%. Similar results were seen in 4S and WOSCOPS, and meta-analyses suggest that statin therapy does reduce stroke (Figure 23).[109,110] In all three trials, treatment with statin reduced the need for coronary bypass surgery and percutaneous transluminal coronary angioplasty (by 27% in CARE; by 37% in 4S and WOSCOPS). MI and other cardiac morbidity were also reduced by statin treatment, as was the need for hospital admissions. In addition to these findings, those from the Post Coronary Artery Bypass Graft (Post-CABG) trial indicate a reduction in the incidence of saphenous vein graft disease and clinical events in stable, post-CABG patients treated with high-dose lovastatin.

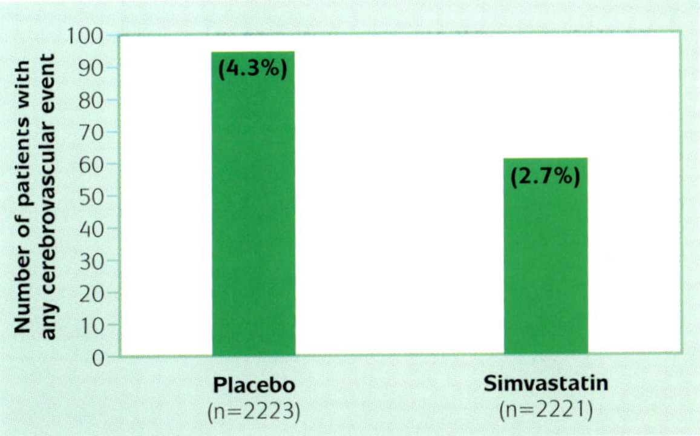

Figure 23. Simvastatin reduced the incidence of stroke compared with placebo in the 4S study. Source: Scandinavian Simvastatin Survival Study Group. *Lancet* 1994;**344**:1383–1389.

At present, the statins are used as first-line lipid-lowering drugs. They reduce LDL-cholesterol, raise HDL-cholesterol and lower triglycerides. Statin drugs do not lower LDL-cholesterol equally well, and differ with regard to their antithrombotic and anti-inflamatory effects.

Preventive Cardiology

Preventive cardiology addresses the prevention of CVD in clinical practice. It focuses on patients with established atherosclerotic disease, the detection and treatment of apparently healthy individuals at high risk of developing CVD, and the families of both groups, especially when there is a history of premature CVD.

The overall aim of preventive cardiology is to reduce the risk of developing symptomatic atherosclerotic disease among apparently healthy high-risk individuals in the general population. In those patients who do develop the disease and survive, the aim is to reduce their risk of recurrent CVD and death. Preventive cardiology therefore aims to improve both quality of life and life expectancy in people at increased risk of developing CVD and patients with established disease.

Clinical settings for preventive cardiology include hospitals (including specialist rehabilitation centres), general or office-based practices, the work place and the private sector.

GPs are in an ideal position to encourage a healthy lifestyle in the community because most people visit their doctor once a year, and doctors are considered to be a credible source of information about the causes of CVD and its prevention. Starting with patients with established atherosclerotic disease, GPs can promote all aspects of prevention and rehabilitation, which inevitably leads to contact with family members who may also be at high risk. In hospitals specialists in hypertension, lipids and diabetes also have the opportunity to advise their patients on healthy lifestyle and to take a multifactorial approach to risk factor assessment and management instead of just focusing on blood pressure, lipids or glucose in isolation. Other specialists (e.g. neurologists, or specialists in peripheral arterial disease or renal disease) have a similar opportunity to broaden their assessment and management of patients with atherosclerotic disease in order to reduce their risk. Opportunistic screening of all patients seen in clinical practice, irrespective of the initial reason for seeking medical advice, will yield even more high-risk individuals for primary prevention.

Although currently the opportunities for physicians to prevent CVD in clinical practice are considerable, this potential is not yet being realized. For patients with established CHD, medical records of risk factors are incomplete and the management of risk factors such as obesity, blood pressure or blood lipids is inadequate compared with recommendations by professional guidelines.[111-113] For many patients with hypertension, or dyslipidaemia or diabetes who have not yet developed CVD, risk factor goals are not being reached. Many GPs do not routinely screen patients with a family history of premature CHD, or check for cardiovascular risk factors in their daily clinical practice. Even when they do so, appropriate action and follow-up are not always taken.

Although the organization of preventive cardiology for coronary patients, high-risk individuals and their families will differ between national medical settings, it is appropriate to define the common principles of care, which are described below for three clinical areas (see Figure 24).

Cardiovascular prevention and rehabilitation

Objective of a cardiovascular prevention and rehabilitation programme

The overall objective in patients who present with symptoms of atherosclerotic CVD (e.g. stable angina, acute coronary syndromes, stroke and peripheral arterial disease) is to slow the progression of the disease and, if possible, induce disease regression and reduce the risk of thrombotic complications. In this way, the risks of a further non-fatal event, or death from CVD, will be reduced and the chances of survival improved. As well as favourably influencing the underlying causes of the disease, it is also important to help create the best physical, mental and social conditions so that patients can lead as full and active a life as possible in society. For the patient, this means a better quality of life and a longer life expectancy.

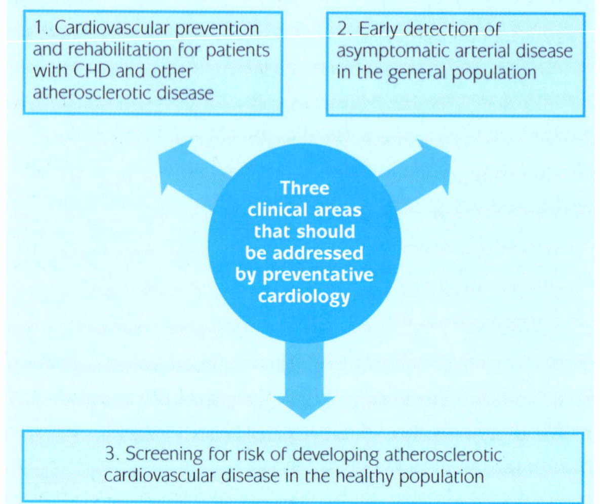

Figure 24. Three clinical areas that should be addressed by preventive cardiology.

Cardiac rehabilitation has its origins in physical rehabilitation, but this specialty has gradually evolved into comprehensive lifestyle programmes (e.g. smoking cessation, making healthy food choices and increasing physical activity) based on behavioural models of change. The following aspects of prevention are now integrated into this approach: risk factor management; controlling blood pressure, lipids and diabetes; and prescribing prophylactic drug therapies such as aspirin, beta-blockers, ACE inhibitors/angiotensin-II receptor blockers and anti-coagulants. Psychosocial and vocational support to help patients lead a full life is also provided. This evolution in cardiac rehabilitation is reflected in the last WHO definition:

The rehabilitation of cardiac patients is the sum of activities required to influence favourably the underlying cause of the disease, as well as the best possible physical, mental and social conditions, so that they may, by their own efforts preserve or resume when lost, as normal a place as possible in the community. Rehabilitation cannot be regarded as an isolated form of therapy but must be integrated with the whole treatment of which it forms only one facet.

Although this definition addresses only cardiac patients, the principles of a cardiovascular prevention programme also apply to patients with other forms of atherosclerotic disease. Patients with cerebrovascular and peripheral atherosclerotic disease have very different physical rehabilitative needs compared with the cardiac patient, but the need for preventive care is the same.

A comprehensive cardiovascular prevention and rehabilitation programme needs a multidisciplinary team of healthcare professionals, including cardiology and other medical specialities, nursing, dietetics, physiotherapy, occupational therapy, pharmacy, health promotion, psychology and behavioural medicine. All of these professions and disciplines have an important contribution to make to a comprehensive prevention and rehabilitation programme for atherosclerotic disease patients and their families.

Content of a cardiovascular prevention and rehabilitation programme

Although the organisation of a cardiovascular prevention and rehabilitation programme varies between different medical settings, there are common components to every programme:

Lifestyle assessment

This includes assessment of smoking, diet and physical activity habits of patients and families.

Risk factor assessment

Assessment of blood pressure, lipids and glycaemia.

Assessment of stage of change

Assessing a patient's stage of change is important and, although there are different behavioural models, DiClemente and Prochaska's "stages of change" is one widely recognized example (Figure25). There are three main stages that the

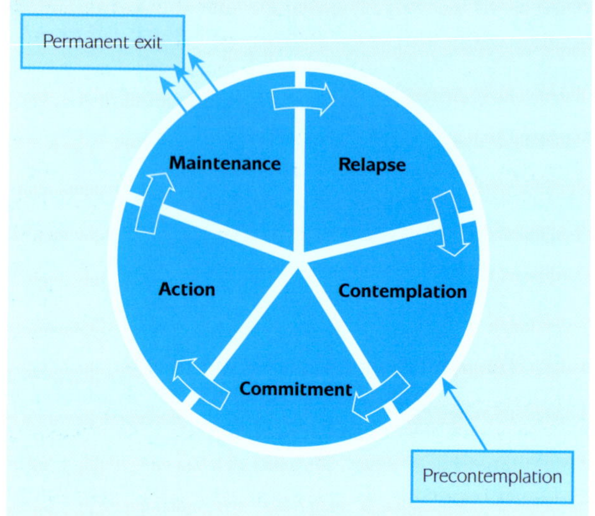

Figure 25. DiClemente's and Prochaska's stages of change.

physician needs to work through with patients. These include preparing and advising the patient to change (the preparation stage), assisting the patient to change (the action stage), and providing the patient with follow-up (the maintenance stage). There is no fixed period required to progress through the stages. While some patients may progress with ease, others may need to be monitored closely during each stage, and others will need to return to an earlier stage after setbacks or relapses. It is important that professionals discuss and negotiate with their patients how best to achieve change.

Health promotion

Promotion of a healthy lifestyle (e.g. avoidance of tobacco use, making healthy food choices and becoming physically active) is the foundation of a prevention and rehabilitation programme. Information needs to be tailored to the patient's needs and level of understanding. Such information should be clear, concrete and specific. Technical terms should be avoided and, where possible, verbal advice should be supplemented with written or audiovisual materials.

Family-based behavioural intervention

To achieve and sustain these lifestyle changes, involvement of the patient's partner and other family members sharing the same household may help. The patient is more likely to quit smoking if their partner is a non- smoker and the whole household is tobacco-free. Dietary changes are more likely to occur if the person responsible for shopping and cooking is involved in the programme, and the whole family makes these changes together. Similarly, for the patient to become more physically active, the role of the family in supporting leisure-time physical activities can also be helpful. The partner and other family members also have to make psychological adjustments to the patient's physical and mental conditions. The sexual relationship between patient and partner is a sensitive and important issue which needs to be addressed. By including the partner in the programme, it is possible for the whole family to come to terms with the illness and then, together, take the necessary steps to reduce the risk of recurrent disease.

Patient education

Patients and families need to be informed about atherosclerotic disease, its causes and how these can be modified, the use of medical and surgical treatments, and cardiopulmonary resuscitation.

Risk factor management

Monitoring is required of risk factors such as weight, body fat distribution, blood pressure, lipids and glucose. Setting risk factor goals (e.g. blood pressure < 140/90 mmHg), and maximizing the doses of drugs in order to achieve them are also required. The Joint European Societies guidelines on blood pressure and lipid management are summarized in Figures 26 and 27.

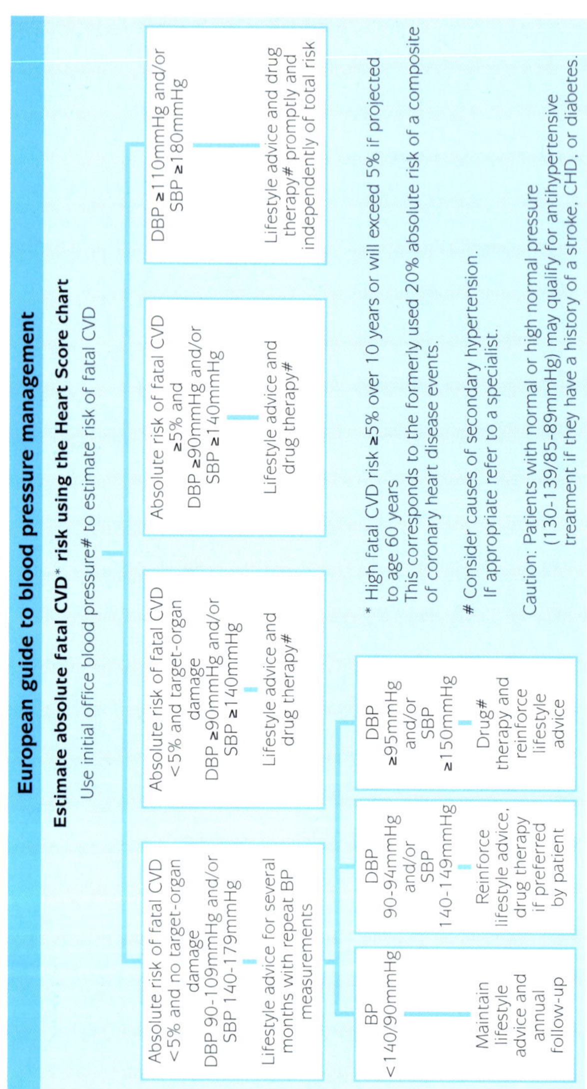

Figure 26. Joint European Society guidelines on blood pressure management. Reproduced with permission from De Backer G *et al. Eur J Cardiovasc Prev Rehabil* 2003;**10**(Suppl. 1):S1–S78.

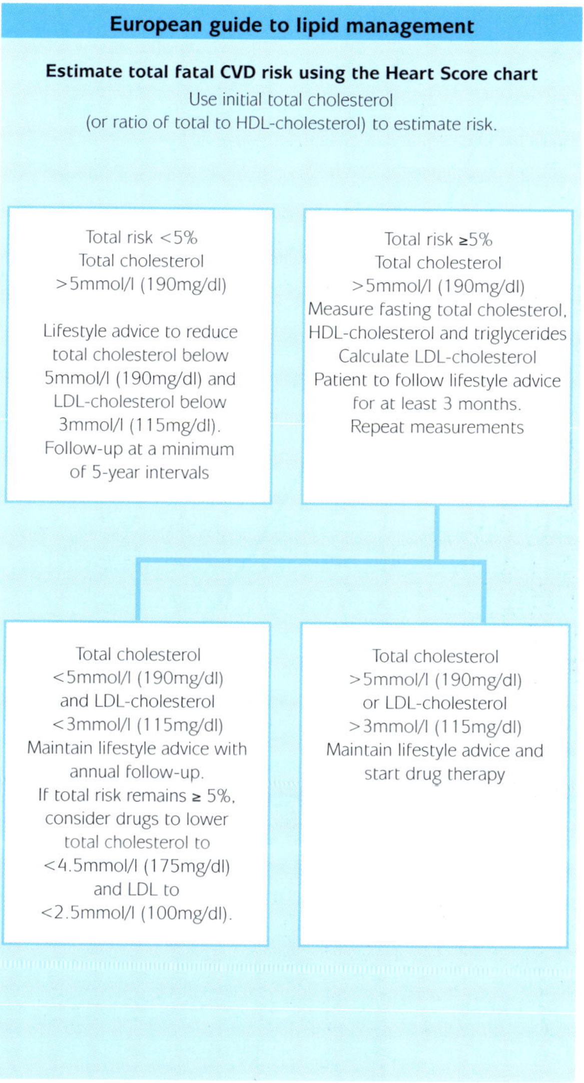

European guide to lipid management

Estimate total fatal CVD risk using the Heart Score chart

Use initial total cholesterol
(or ratio of total to HDL-cholesterol) to estimate risk.

Total risk <5%
Total cholesterol
>5mmol/l (190mg/dl)

Lifestyle advice to reduce total cholesterol below 5mmol/l (190mg/dl) and LDL-cholesterol below 3mmol/l (115mg/dl).
Follow-up at a minimum of 5-year intervals

Total risk ≥5%
Total cholesterol
>5mmol/l (190mg/dl)
Measure fasting total cholesterol, HDL-cholesterol and triglycerides
Calculate LDL-cholesterol
Patient to follow lifestyle advice for at least 3 months.
Repeat measurements

Total cholesterol
<5mmol/l (190mg/dl)
and LDL-cholesterol
<3mmol/l (115mg/dl)
Maintain lifestyle advice with annual follow-up.
If total risk remains ≥ 5%, consider drugs to lower total cholesterol to <4.5mmol/l (175mg/dl) and LDL to <2.5mmol/l (100mg/dl).

Total cholesterol
>5mmol/l (190mg/dl)
or LDL-cholesterol
>3mmol/l (115mg/dl)
Maintain lifestyle advice and start drug therapy

Figure 27. Joint European Society guidelines on lipid management. Reproduced with permission from De Backer G *et al. Eur J Cardiovasc Prev Rehabil* 2003;**10**(Suppl. 1):S1–S78.

Drug therapies and patient compliance

Drugs will be required in some patients to control blood pressure, lipids and glycaemia. In addition, some drugs such as aspirin, beta-blockers and ACE inhibitors/angiotensin-II receptor blockers and anticoagulants are given prophylactically. When a drug is prescribed, it is important to ensure, wherever possible, that the dose is that used in clinical trials that have demonstrated efficacy and safety of such treatments.

Psychological issues

The emotional responses to the development of CVD and how these can be addressed need to be understood if the patient is to be able to take the necessary steps through lifestyle changes to reduce the risk of recurrent disease. Stress management and relaxation are part of this process.

Screening of first-degree blood relatives

Patients with premature CHD, men under 55 years and women under 65 years should have their immediate blood relatives screened for cardiovascular risk factors: parents (if appropriate), siblings and offspring. For the patient's younger children (< 18 years old), smoking, body weight and physical activity need to be addressed but screening of blood pressure, lipids and glucose can be deferred until adulthood unless familial hypercholesterolaemia is suspected.

Vocational issues

Professional advice and help in making the necessary preparations to return to work, or seek alternative work, is important if the patient is to resume as full a role in society as they wish. Licensing implications for driving will also have to be considered.

Quality assurance of preventive cardiology programme

Whatever the content of a cardiovascular prevention and rehabilitation programme, it is essential to audit the whole process and outcome of care. Based on practical experience, a programme can only evolve and achieve its stated objectives through auditing of the following parameters: characteristics of patients who take up and adhere to the programme, compared with those who do not; prevalence of lifestyle and other risk factors at entry to the programme; lifestyle changes and the levels of blood pressure, cholesterol, etc, achieved by the end of the programme; proportions of patients (and families) achieving the recommended national lifestyle, risk factor and therapeutic goals.

Early detection of atherosclerotic arterial disease in the healthy population

As sudden cardiac collapse and death can be the first manifestation of CVD, the impetus to detect atherosclerotic disease earlier in its asymptomatic phase is considerable. Sudden death is not the only incentive for early disease detection. Some patients may survive their first clinical presentation of atherosclerotic disease, but be so severely disabled that prevention and rehabilitation has very little to offer.

Principles of screening for asymptomatic disease

Objective of screening programme

The objective of an atherosclerotic disease detection programme is to identify those who have asymptomatic disease among apparently healthy individuals in the general population in order to slow the progression of the disease, induce regression if possible, and also reduce the risk of thrombotic complications. In this way, the risk of a first non-fatal or fatal cardiovascular event can be postponed or even prevented.

The medical technology to detect atherosclerotic arterial disease and its clinical sequelae is already available, but its role in population screening has yet to be evaluated.

A screening test for coronary artery disease, or other atherosclerotic disease, has to meet a number of criteria before it can be used in the general population. These criteria include:

- The non-invasive technique for detecting atherosclerotic disease is valid, precise, easy and acceptable.
- The relationship between atherosclerotic disease detected non-invasively and the development of symptomatic disease such as angina or MI, stroke or cardiovascular death has been quantified.
- There is defined screening strategy.
- Trained staff and facilities for screening and intervention are available.
- There is a defined intervention and follow-up policy.
- Screening and intervention results in a reduction in clinical events such as cardiovascular morbidity and mortality.
- Screening has no adverse effects.
- The cost of screening and intervention is justified in relation to the outcome.

For the individual being screened for atherosclerotic disease there are three questions to ask (Table 25). In other words, will the individual's quality and quantity of life be both improved.

Techniques for the detection of symptomatic disease

Several techniques are in development or in clinical use for the detection of asymptomatic disease. These include: magnetic resonance imaging (MRI) for coronary or other atherosclerotic plaques; electron beam computed tomography (EBCT) or multi-slice CT (MSCT) for coronary calcified atherosclerosis; and ultrasound of the carotids and other major peripheral arteries for atherosclerotic disease. MRI is still in the research phase but EBCT, which measures the amount of coronary calcification expressed as an Agatston score, is being used in selected clinical settings.

The Agatston score is a measure of the burden of coronary artery disease and also its prognosis, and these relationships are independent of classic risk factors. Calcium scanning can therefore further refine risk assessment of an asymptomatic individual, but its role in

Screening for atherosclerotic disease
1. Will I feel any better?
2. Will my risk of developing symptomatic disease and its complications be reduced?
3. Will I live longer?

Table 25. Three questions an individual should ask to determine the benefits of a general population screening programme for atherosclerotic arterial disease.

clinical practice is still being evaluated. Ultrasound of the peripheral arteries is a well-established imaging modality in clinical practice. Carotid ultrasound measures intima–media thickness (IMT) and plaque characteristics: as IMT increases so does the risk of cardiovascular disease, both cerebral and coronary events, which is independent of other risk factors.

At present non-invasive methods for the detection of asymptomatic atherosclerotic disease are rapidly evolving, but more research is needed to evaluate the role of MRI and EBCT in clinical practice. Clinical trials are required to evaluate the impact of a non-invasive screening programme for atherosclerotic disease on subsequent cardiovascular morbidity and mortality, compared with conventional risk factor screening of the healthy population. Population-screening programmes to detect asymptomatic arterial disease are currently not justified.

Screening for cardiovascular risk factors in the healthy population

Screening the healthy population for risk of developing CVD is necessary in order to identify and target apparently healthy but high-risk individuals for lifestyle and, where appropriate, therapeutic interventions.

Objective of a cardiovascular screening programme

The overall objective of a cardiovascular screening programme is therefore to detect and treat high-risk individuals in order to reduce the risk of a first non-fatal or fatal cardiovascular event.

Principles of risk factor screening

Mass screening of the whole adult population is not required as there are other ways through existing medical services to identify and treat such high-risk individuals. Screening for risk factors can only be justified if the criteria already defined for early disease detection are met. These are summarized in Table 26.

There is compelling scientific evidence for unifactorial interventions in relation to smoking, blood pressure, blood lipids, etc., which has laid the foundation for multi-factorial screening and prevention programmes. However, such programmes must be able to bring about the same risk factor changes achieved in the unifactorial trials and, if this is accomplished, there will be a reduction in CVD.

Screening can be undertaken systematically, in all middle-aged adults living in one community, for example, or opportunistically, in people making contact with the medical system irrespective of their reason for doing so. Such opportunities can be used to assess and act upon cardiovascular

Criteria for justifying risk factor screening

- There is a defined screening and intervention strategy
- The interventions have been shown to reduce the risk of clinical events such as cardiovascular morbidity and mortality
- The cost of screening and intervention is justified in relation to the outcome

Table 26. Criteria that must be met in order to justify screening for cardiovascular risk factors.

risk factors. Whether systematic or opportunistic, the act of screening is a commitment by the health professional to give lifestyle advice, make follow-up measurements and undertake appropriate investigations such as laboratory tests.

All adults are potentially eligible for cardiovascular screening, but uncritical cardiovascular screening for every adult is inappropriate. In younger adults, under the age of 40 years, some aspects of lifestyle are particularly important: smoking, obesity, sedentary existence, alcohol consumption and, for women, the use of oral contraceptives and their potential cardiovascular complications. Lifestyle counselling maybe all that is required at this age, although a small minority will have hypertension, dyslipidaemia or diabetes requiring drug treatment.

While lifestyle continues to be important in middle life (40–69 years old), the physiological and metabolic consequences, in terms of hypertension, dyslipidaemia and diabetes, become more common, and an increasing proportion of this section of the population therefore has individually high-risk factors. A multifactorial fatal CVD risk greater or equal to 5% over 10 years in Europe justifies intensive lifestyle and, where necessary, therapeutic interventions. For women, a premature menopause either natural or surgically induced, in particular if the latter case is associated with removal of the ovaries, increases the risk of premature CHD. Particular attention to lifestyle and other cardiovascular risk factors in such women is therefore important.

The largest proportion of high-risk individuals is found in the older population (≥ 70 years old), and systolic hypertension will be a particularly common problem. However, because of significant comorbidity in this group, clinical judgement is required when making decisions on specific screening for cardiovascular risk factors. Many of these individuals are at higher absolute CVD risk than any other section of the population, and are therefore potentially more likely to benefit from risk factor reductions, in particular SBP and cholesterol. However, evidence for some risk factor interventions, in particular in the very elderly, is not available and judgement is again required on what action, if any, to take.

From the information above, screening for multifactorial risk is inevitably focused on middle-aged individuals, in whom risk factors are common and evidence of benefit from interventions is most secure.

Content of a cardiovascular screening and intervention programme

While the organisation of a cardiovascular screening programme inevitably varies between different medical settings, it is possible to define the main contents common to such programmes (Table 27). All of these subjects have been addressed earlier.

Evaluation of the process, and of lifestyle and risk factor management outcomes, is necessary in order to inform the physician and other health professionals on the success of the intervention, and how it can be improved.

Key features of cardiovasular screening programmes
• Lifestyle and cardiovascular risk assessment • Behavioural change • Health promotion • Education • Family-based intervention • Risk factor management • Screening of first-degree blood relatives where appropriate

Table 27. Key features of cardiovascular screening programmes.

Future developments

Development of risk assessment

As knowledge of epidemiological, clinical and basic sciences increases, so does our understanding of the causes and mechanisms of CVD. It will therefore be possible to refine risk assessment to better identify those individuals who are at increased risk of developing or having recurrent CVD. New risk factors are being recognized and evaluated including markers of inflammation, and thrombogenic and genetic factors. Such knowledge will also lead to new forms of lifestyle and therapeutic interventions leading to more effective risk reduction.

Gene therapy

With the advent of the human genome project, and genetic, molecular and cellular technology, cardiovascular medicine is now on the threshold of an era of increased understanding of both the causes of CVD and the potential for genetically tailored therapies. The concept of gene therapy encompasses a broad range of diverse techniques having as a common aim the transfer and expression of specific genes that have potential therapeutic value.

Frequently asked questions

What is atherosclerosis?

Atherosclerosis is the build-up of fatty substances, collectively called atheroma, within the walls of arteries.

What is coronary heart disease?

Coronary heart disease is a common term to describe atherosclerosis of the arteries that supply the heart muscle with blood and oxygen. The coronary arteries become diseased with fatty deposits called atheroma. Atheroma of the coronary arteries can cause angina, heart attack or sudden death.

What is angina pectoris?

Angina is pain in the chest, usually brought on by exertion or emotion. The pain is caused by a reduction in blood flow to the heart muscle. This is due to a narrowing of the coronary arteries with fatty deposits called atheroma. You may feel the pain in your chest or between your shoulders, or in your arms, jaw or throat. If you have chest pain you should consult your doctor.

What is a heart attack?

A heart attack happens when one of the coronary arteries suddenly becomes blocked by a blood clot. This blockage completely stops the blood supply to that part of the heart muscle which it serves, which usually causes severe pain in the centre of the chest. If you think you are having a heart attack you should call the emergency medical service and take one tablet of aspirin.

My father died of a heart attack when he was 45 years. Am I at increased risk of a heart attack?

Yes. When heart disease develops at a younger age – in men aged under 55 years and in women under 65 years – the immediate relatives of these patients may be at increased risk of heart disease. If you have a family history of premature heart disease you should consult your doctor.

Can I change any of my existing risk factors for coronary heart disease?

Yes, the risk factors that you can change are: smoking, unhealthy eating habits, being physically inactive, being overweight, high blood pressure, high cholesterol and diabetes. You may need the help of a doctor and other health professionals to make lifestyle changes and control other risk factors.

I have been smoking for over 10 years. Is there any benefit in stopping now or is it too late?

Yes, quitting smoking will decrease your risk of developing coronary heart disease in future.

How may I improve my diet?

You have to eat less fat and replace saturated fat with monounsaturated and polyunsaturated fat (for example, use rapeseed, olive or sunflower oil); increase the amount of fish you eat; eat more fruit and vegetables (at least five portions a day); and eat more fibre (for example beans, peas, lentils and oats).

Does fish consumption improve the prognosis after myocardial infarction?

Yes. Fish consumption reduces mortality after myocardial infarction and the same is true for fish oil capsules.

Is alcohol good for heart disease?

Where there are no contraindications to alcohol use, 10–30 g of ethanol per day for men and 10–20 g of ethanol per day for women may be considered safe.

How much do I need to exercise?

You need to exercise frequently and regularly. For the healthy population the target is a total of 30–45 minutes' moderate activity a day, four to five times weekly.

What types of physical activity should I do?

Some of the best types of activity are walking, cycling, dancing and everyday activities such as climbing the stairs. The exercise must not cause you any pain.

What are cardioprotective drug therapies?

Several classes of drugs, including antiplatelet therapies, beta-blockers, ACE inhibitors/angiotensin-II receptor blockers, lipid-modification therapies and anticoagulants, can reduce the risk of developing or having recurrent cardiovascular disease.

How long do I have to take such cardioprotective drugs?

In general, cardioprotective drugs are prescribed for the lifetime of the patient.

References

1. Murray C J L, Lopez A D. Mortality by cause for eight regions of the world: Global Burden of Disease Study. *Lancet* 1997;**349**:1269–1276.

2. Murray C J L, Lopez A D. Alternative projections of mortality and disability by cause 1990–2020: Global Burden of Disease Study. *Lancet* 1997;**349**:1498–1504.

3. Levi F, Lucchini F, Negri E *et al*. Trends in mortality from cardiovascular and cerebrovascular diseases in Europe and other areas of the world. *Heart* 2002;**88**:119–124.

4. Bartechi CE, MacKenzie TD, Schrier RW. The human costs of tobacco use (first of two parts). *N Engl J Med* 1994;**330**:907–912.

5. MacKenzie TD, Bartechi CE, Schrier RW. The human costs of tobacco use (second of two parts). *N Engl J Med* 1994; **330**:975–980.

6. Dwyer JH. Exposure to environmental tobacco smoke and coronary risk. *Circulation* 1997;**96**:1403–1407.

7. Liam TH, He Y. Passive smoking and coronary heart disease: a brief review. *Clin Exp Pharmacol Physiol* 1997;**24**:993–996.

8. Law MR, Morris JK, Wald NJ. Environmental tobacco smoke exposure and ischaemic heart disease: an evaluation of the evidence. *BMJ* 1997;**315**:973–982.

9. World Health Organization. Diet, nutrition and prevention of chronic diseases. Report of a WHO Study Group. WHO Technical Report Series 797. Geneva: World Health Organization, 1990.

10. Hu FB, Manson JE, Willett WC. Types of dietary fat and the risk of coronary heart disease: a critical review. *J Amer Col Nutr* 2001;**20**:5–19.

11. Brousseau ME, Schafer EJ. Diet and coronary heart disease: clinical trials. *Cur Atheroscl Reports* 2000;**2**:487–493.

12. Rosengren A, Wilhemsen L. Physical activity protects against coronary death and death from all causes in middle-aged men. Evidence from a 20-year follow-up of the primary prevention study in Göteborg. *Ann Epidemiol* 1997;**7**:69–75.

13. Folsom AR, Arnett DK, Hutchinson RG *et al*. Physical activity and incidence of coronary heart disease in middle-aged women and men. *Med Sci Sports Exerc* 1997;**29**:901–909.

14. Wannamethee SG, Shaper AG. Physical activity in the prevention of cardiovascular disease: an epidemiological perspective. *Sports Medicine* 2001;**31**:101–114.

15. Leon AS, Myers MT, Connett J. Leisure time physical activity and the 16 year risks of mortality from coronary heart disease and all causes in the multiple risk factor intervention trial (MRFIT). *Int J Sports Med* 1997;**18**(Suppl. 3):208–215.

16. Blair SN, Kampert JB, Kohl HW *et al*. Influences of cardiorespiratory fitness and other precursors on cardiovascular disease and all cause mortality in men and women. *JAMA* 1996; **276**:205–210.

17. Sesso HD, Paffenbarger RS, Jr, Lee IM. Physical activity and coronary heart disease in men: The Harvard Alumni Health Study. *Circulation* 2000;**102**(9):975–980.

18. Larsson B. Obesity and body fat distribution as predictors of coronary heart disease. In: Marmot M, Elliott P, eds. *Coronary heart disease epidemiology. From aetiology to public health*. Oxford: Oxford University Press, 1992.

19. Rimm EB, Stampfer MJ, Giovannucci E *et al*. Body size and fat distribution as predictors of coronary heart disease among middle-aged and older US men. *Am J Epidemiol* 1995; **141**:1117–1127.

20. Prineas RJ, Folsom AR, Kaye SA. Central adiposity and increased risk of coronary mortality in older women. *Ann Epidemiol* 1993;**3**:35–41.

21. Folsom AR, Kaye SA, Sellers TA *et al*. Body fat distribution and 5-year risk of death in older women. *JAMA* 1993; **269**:483–487.

22. Rimm EB, Williams P, Fosher K *et al*. Moderate alcohol intake and lower risk of coronary heart disease: meta-analysis of effects on lipids and haemostatic factors. *BMJ* 1999; **319**:1523–1528.

23. Royal College of Physicians. Report of a Joint Working Group of the Royal College of Physicians, Psychiatrists and General Practitioners. Alcohol and heart in perspective. London: Royal College of Physicians, 1995.

24. McMahon R, Peto R, Cuttler J *et al*. Blood pressure, stroke and coronary heart disease. Part 1. Prolonged differences in blood pressure: prospective observational studies corrected for the regression dilution bias. *Lancet* 1990;**335**:765–774.

25. Kannel WB. Blood pressure as a cardiovascular risk factor: prevention and treatment. *JAMA* 1996;**275**:1571–1576.

26. Walker WG, Neaton JD, Cutler JA *et al*. Renal function change in hypertensive members of the Multiple Risk Factor Intervention Trial. Racial and treatment effects. The MRFIT Research Group. *JAMA* 1992;**268**:3085–3091.

27. Neaton JD, Blackburn H, Jacobs D *et al*. Serum cholesterol level and mortality findings for men screened in the Multiple Risk Factor Intervention Trial. *Arch Intern Med* 1992;**152**:1490–1500.

28 Davey-Smith G, Shipley MJ, Marmot MG *et al*. Plasma cholesterol and mortality: The Whitehall Study. *JAMA* 1992;**267**:70–76.

29. Chen Z, Peto R, Collins R *et al*. Serum cholesterol concentration and coronary heart disease in a population with low cholesterol concentrations. *Br Med J* 1991;**303**:276–282.

30. Hokanson JE, Austin MA. Plasma triglyceride level is a risk factor for cardiovascular disease independent of high-density lipoprotein cholesterol level: a meta-analysis of population-based prospective studies. *J Cardiovasc Risk* 1996;**3**:213–219.

31. Austin MA. Triacylglycerol and coronary heart disease. *Proc Nutr Soc* 1997;**56**:667–670.

32. Cullen P. Evidence that triglycerides are an independent coronary heart disease risk factor. *Am J Cardiol* 2000;**86**:943–949.

33. Goldbourt U, Yaari S, Medalie JH. Isolated low HDL cholesterol as a risk factor for coronary heart disease mortality: a 21-year follow-up of 8000 men. *Atheroscler Thromb Vasc Biol* 1997;**17**:107–113.

34. Khaw KT, Wareham N, Luben R *et al*. Glycated haemoglobin, diabetes, and mortality in men in Norfolk cohort of European prospective investigation of cancer and nutrition (EPIC- Norfolk). *BMJ* 2001;**322**:15–18.

35. Glucose tolerance and mortality: comparison of WHO and American Diabetes Association diagnostic criteria. The DECODE study group. European Diabetes Epidemiology Group. Diabetes Epidemiology: Collaborative analysis Of Diagnostic criteria in Europe. *Lancet* 1999;**354**:617–621.

36. World Health Organization. Definition, diagnosis and classification of diabetes mellitus and its complications. Report of a WHO consultation. Part 1: diagnosis and classification of diabetes mellitus. WHO/NCD/NCS/99.2. Geneva: World Health Organization, 1999.

37. The Expert Committee on the diagnosis and classification of diabetes mellitus. Report of the Expert Committee on the diagnosis and classification of diabetes mellitus. *Diabetes Care* 2002;**25**:S5–S20.

38. American Diabetes Association. Standards of medical care for patients with diabetes mellitus. *Diabetes Care* 2003;**26**(Suppl. 1): S33–S50.

39. European Diabetes Policy Group 1998. A desktop guide to Type 1 (insulin-dependent) diabetes mellitus. *Diabetic Medicine* 1999:**16**:253–266.

40. European Diabetes Policy Group 1999. A desktop guide to Type 2 diabetes mellitus. *Diabetic Medicine* 1999;**16**:716–730.

41. Haffner SM, Miettinen H. Insulin resistance implications for type II diabetes mellitus and coronary heart disease. *Am J Med* 1997;**103**:152–162.

42. Ford ES, Giles WH, Dietz WH. Prevalence of the metabolic syndrome among US adults: findings from the third National Health and Nutrition Examination Survey. *JAMA* 2002;**287**:356–359.

43. Laakso M. Insulin resistance and coronary heart disease. *Curr Opin Lipidol* 1996;**7**:217–226.

44. Ford ES, Smith SJ, Stroup DF *et al*. Homocyst(e)ine and cardiovascular disease: a systematic review of the evidence with special emphasis on case-control studies and nested case-control studies. *Int J Epidemiol* 2002;**31**:59–70.

45. Libby P, Ridker PM, Maseri A. Inflammation and atherosclerosis. *Circulation* 2002;**105**:1135–1143.

46. Danesh J. Is there a link between chronic Helicobacter pylory infection and coronary heart disease? *Eur J Surgery* 1998; **Suppl.**(582):27–31.

47. Sesso HD, Lee IM, Gaziano M *et al*. Maternal and paternal history of myocardial infarction and risk of cardiovascular disease in men and women. *Circulation* 2001;**104**:393–398.

48. Anderson KM, Wilson PWF, Odell PM *et al*. An updated coronary risk profile: A statement for health professionals. *Circulation* 1991;**83**:356–362.

49. Jackson R, Barham P, Bills J *et al*. Management of raised blood pressure in New Zealand: a discussion document. *BMJ* 1993;**307**:107-110.

50. National Heart Foundation. Clinical Guidelines for the assessment and management of dyslipidaemia. *NZ Med J* 1996;**109**:224–232.

51. Jackson R. Updated New Zealand cardiovascular disease risk-benefit prediction guide. *BMJ* 2000;**320**:709–710.

52. Pyörälä K, De Backer G, Graham I *et al*. Prevention of coronary heart disease in clinical practice. Recommendations of the Task Force of the European Society of Cardiology, European Atherosclerotic Society and European Society of Hypertension. *Eur Heart J* 1994;**15**:1300–1331.

53. Wood D, De Backer G, Faergeman O *et al*. Prevention of coronary heart disease in clinical practice. Recommendations of the Second Joint Task Force of European and other Societies on coronary prevention. *Eur Heart J* 1998;**19**:1434–1503.

54. De Backer G, Ambrosioni E, Borch-Johnsen K *et al*. European guidelines on cardiovascular disease prevention in clinical practice. Executive Summary. Third Joint Task Force of European and other Societies on Cardiovascular Disease Prevention in Clinical Practice (constituted by representatives of eight societies

and by invited experts). *Eur J Cardiovasc Prev Rehabil* 2003;**10**:S1–S10; *Eur Heart J* 2003;**24**:1604–1610.

55. Joint British recommendations on prevention of coronary heart disease in clinical practice: summary. British Cardiac Society, British Hyperlipidaemia Association, British Hypertension Society, British Diabetic Association. *BMJ* 2000;**320**:705–708.

56. Wood DA, Durrington P, Poulter N *et al*. on behalf of British Cardiac Society, British Hyperlipidaemia Association, British Hypertension Society, British Diabetic Association. Joint British recommendations on prevention of coronary heart disease in clinical practice. *Heart* 1998; **80**(Suppl. 2):S1–S29.

57. Haq IU, Jackson PR, Yeo WW *et al*. Sheffield risk and treatment table for cholesterol lowering for primary prevention of coronary heart disease. *Lancet* 1995;**346**:1467–1471.

58. Wallis EJ, Ramsay LE, Haq IU *et al*. Coronary and cardiovascular risk estimation for primary prevention: validation of a new Sheffield table in the 1995 Scotish health survey population. *BMJ* 2000;**320**:671–676.

59. National Institutes of Health. Third Report of the National Cholesterol Education Program (NCEP) Expert Panel on Detection, Evaluation, and Treatment of High Blood Cholesterol in Adults (Adult Treatment Panel III). Executive Summary. NIH Publication No 01-3670. Bethesda: National Institues of Health, May 2001.

60. Haq IU, Ramsay LE, Yeo WW *et al*. Is the Framingham risk function valid for northern European populations? A comparison of methods for estimating absolute coronary risk in high risk men. *Heart* 1999;**81**:40–46.

61. Pyorala K. Assessment of coronary heart disease risk in populations with different levels of risk. *Eur Heart J* 2000; **21**:348–350.

62. Conroy RM, Pyorala K, Fitzgerald AP *et al*. Estimation of ten-year risk of fatal cardiovascular disease in Europe: the SCORE project. *Eur Hear J* 2003;**24**:987–1003.

63. Ramsay LE, Williams B, Johnston GE *et al*. British Hypertension Society guidelines for hypertension management 1999: summary. *BMJ* 1999;**319**:630–635.

64. Ramsay L, Williams B, Johnston G *et al*. Guidelines for management of hypertension: report of the Third working party of the British Hypertension Society. *J Hum Hypertens* 1999; **13**:569–592.

65. The Seventh Report of the Joint National Committee on Prevention, Detection, Evaluation, and Treatment of High Blood Pressure. The JNC 7 Report. *JAMA* 2003;**289**:2560–2572.

66. Raw M, McNeil A, West R. Smoking cessation guidelines for health professionals. A guide to effective smoking cessation inventions for the health care system. *Thorax* 1998;**53**(Suppl. 5): S1–S38.

67. A clinical practice guideline for treating tobacco use and dependence. A US Public Health Service Report. *JAMA* 2000; **283**:3244–3254.

68. Balfour D, Benowitz N, Fagerström K *et al*. Diagnosis and treatment of nicotine dependence with emphasis on nicotine replacement therapy. *Eur Heart J* 2000;**21**:438–445.

69. Giannuzzi P, Mezzani A, Saner H *et al*. Physical activity for primary and secondary prevention. Position paper of the Working Group on Cardiac Rehabilitation and Exercise Physiology of the European Society of Cardiology. *Eur J Cardiovasc Prevention Rehabilitation* 2003;**10**:319–327.

70. Balady G, Ades P, Bazzarre T *et al*. Core components of cardiac rehabilitation/secondary prevention programs. Statement for healthcare professionals from the American Heart Association and the American Association of Cardiovascular and Pulmonary Rehabilitation. *Circulation* 2000;**102**:1069–1073.

71. Fletcher G for the Task Force on Risk Reduction. How to implement physical activity in primary and secondary prevention. A statement for healthcare professionals from the Task Force on risk reduction, American Heart Association. *Circulation* 1997;**96**: 355–357.

72. Anderson JW, Konz EC. Obesity and disease management: effects of weight loss on comorbid conditions. *Obes Res* 2001;**9**(Suppl. 4):326S–334S.

73. Luque CA, Rey JA. Sibutramine: a serotonin-norepinephrine reuptake-inhibitor for the treatment of obesity. *Ann Pharmacother* 1999;**33**:968–978.

74. Bhatt DL, Topol EJ. Antiplatelet and anticoagulant therapy in the secondary prevention of ischemic heart disease. *Med Clin North Am* 2000;**84**:163–179.

75. Antiplatelet Trialist's Collaboration. Collaborative meta-anlysis of randomized trials of antiplatelet therapy for prevention of death, myocardial infarction, and stroke in high risk patients. *BMJ* 2002;**324**:71–86.

76. Aronow WS. Antiplatelet agents in the prevention of cardiovascular morbidity and mortality in older patients with vascular disease. *Drugs Aging* 1999;**15**:91–101.

77. Hennekens CH, Dyken ML, Fuster V. Aspirin as a therapeutic agent in cardiovascular disease. A statement for Healthcare Professionals from the American Heart Association. *Circulation* 1997;**96**:2751–2753.

78. Eccles M, Freemantle N, Mason J and the North of England Aspirin Guideline Development Group. North of England evidence based guideline development project: guideline on the use of aspirin as secondary prophylaxis for vascular disease in primary care. *BMJ* 1998;**316**:1303–1309.

79. Hansson L, Zanchettti A, Carruthers SG *et al*. for the HOT study group. Effects of intensive blood pressure lowering and low-dose aspirin in patients with hypertension: principal results to the Hypertension Optimal Study (HOT) randomised trial. *Lancet* 1998;**351**:1755–1762.

80. The Medical Research council's General Practice Research Framework. Thrombosis Prevention Trial: randomised trial of low-intensity oral anticoagulation with warfarin and low-dose aspirin in the primary prevention of ischaemic heart disease in men at increased risk. *Lancet* 1998;**351**:233–241.

81. Sanmuganathan PS, Ghahramani P, Jackson PR *et al*. Aspirin for primary prevention of coronary heart disease: safety and absolute benefit related to coronary risk derived from meta-analysis of randomised trials. *Heart* 2001;**85**:265–271.

82. Bertrand ME, Rupprecht HJ, Urban P *et al*. Double-blind study of the safety of clopidogrel with and without a loading dose in combination with aspirin compared with ticlodipine in combination with aspirin after coronary stending: the clopidogrel

aspirin international cooperative study (CLASSICS). *Circulation* 2000;**102**:624–649.

83. CAPRIE Steering Committee. A randomised, blinded, trial of clopidogrel versus aspirin in patients at risk of ischaemic events (CAPRIE). *Lancet* 1996;**348**:1329–1339.

84. Anand SS, Yusuf S. Oral anticoagulant therapy in patients with coronary artery disease: a meta-analysis. *JAMA* 1999; **282**:2058–2067.

85. Smith P. Oral anticoagulants are effective long-term after acute myocardial infarction. *J Intern Med* 1999;**245**:383–387.

86. Freemantle N, Cleland J, Young P *et al*. β-blockade after myocardial infarction: systematic review and meta regression analysis. *BMJ* 1999;**318**:1730–1737.

87. Gottlieb SS, McCarter RJ, Vogel RA. Effects of beta-blockade on mortality among high-risk and low-risk patients after myocardial infarction. *NEJM* 1998;**339**:489–497.

88. Soriano JB, Hoes AW, Meems L *et al*. Increased survival with beta-blockers: importance of ancillary properties. *Prog Cardiovasc Dis* 1997;**39**:445–456.

89. Lee S, Spencer A. Beta-blockers to reduce mortality in patients with systolic dysfunction: a meta-analysis. *J Fami Pract* 2001;**50**:499–504.

90. Aronow WS. Postinfarction use of beta-blockers in elderly patients. *Drugs Aging* 1997;**11**:424–432.

91. Frishman WH, Cheng A. Secondary prevention of myocardial infarction: role of beta-adrenergic blockers and angiotensin-converting enzyme inhibitors. *Am Heart J* 1999;**137**:S25–S34.

92. Tendera M, Ochala A. Overview of the results of recent beta-blocker trials. *Curr Opin Cardiol* 2001;**16**:180–185.

93. Vantrimpont P, Rouleau JL, Wun CC *et al*. Additive beneficial effects of beta-blockers to angiotensin-converting enzyme inhibitors in the Survival and Ventricular Enlargement (SAVE) Study. SAVE Investigators. *J Am Coll Cardiol* 1997;**29**:229–236.

94. ACE-inhibitor Myocardial Infarction Collaborative Group. Indications for ACE-inhibitors in the early treatment of acute myocardial infarction: systematic overview of individual data

from 100,000 patients in randomised trials. *Circulation* 1998;**97**:2202–2212.

95. Domanski MJ, Exner DV, Borkowf CB *et al*. Effect of angiotensin converting enzyme inhibition on sudden cardiac death in patients following acute myocardial infarction. A meta-analysis of randomized clinical trials. *JACC* 1999;**33**:598–604.

96. Yusuf S, Lonn E. Anti-ischaemic effects of ACE inhibitors: review of current clinical evidence and ongoing clinical trials. *Eur Heart J* 1998;**19**(Suppl. J):J36–J44.

97. Sleight P. Angiotensin II and trials of cardiovascular outcomes. *Am J Cardiol* 2002;**89**:11A–16A.

98. Yusuf S, Sleight P, Pogue J *et al*. Effects of an angiotensin-converting-enzyme inhibitor, ramipril, on cardiovascular events in high-risk patients. The Heart Outcomes Prevention Evaluation Study Investigators. *N Engl J Med* 2000;**342**:145–153.

99. Fox KM. EURopean trial On reduction of cardiac events with Perindopril in stable coronary Artery disease Investigators. Efficacy of perindopril in reduction of cardiovascular events among patients with stable coronary artery disease: randomised, double-blind, placebo-controlled, multicentre trial (the EUROPA study). *Lancet* 2003;**362**:782–788.

100. Dahlof B. Devereux RB. Kjeldsen SE *et al*. The LIFE Study Group. Cardiovascular morbidity and mortality in the Losartan Intervention For Endpoint reduction in hypertension study (LIFE): a randomised trial against atenolol. *Lancet* 2002;**359**:995–1003.

101. Lindholm LH, Ibsen H, Dahlof B *et al*. The LIFE Study Group.Cardiovascular morbidity and mortality in patients with diabetes in the Losartan Intervention For Endpoint reduction in hypertension study (LIFE): a randomised trial against atenolol. *Lancet* 2002;**359**:1004–1010.

102. Brenner BM, Cooper ME, de Zeeuw D *et al*. Effects of losartan on renal and cardiovascular outcomes in patients with type 2 diabetes and nephropathy. *N Engl J Med* 2001; **345**:861–869.

103. Scandinavian Simvastatin Survival Study Group. Randomised trial of cholesterol lowering in 4444 patients with coronary heart disease: the Scandinavian simvastatin survival study. *Lancet* 1994;**344**:1383–1389.

104. Sacks FM, Pfeffer MA, Moye LA *et al*. The effect of pravastatin on coronary events after myocardial infarction in patients with average cholesterol levels. *N Engl J Med* 1996; **335**:1001–1009.

105. The Long-Term Intervention with Pravastatin in Ischaemic Disease (LIPID) Study Group. Prevention of cardiovascular events and death with pravastatin in patients with coronary heart disease and a broad range of initial cholesterol levels. *N Engl J Med* 1998;**339**:1349–1357.

106. Shepherd J, Cobbe SM, Ford I *et al*. Prevention of coronary heart disease with pravastatin in men with hypercholesterolemia. West of Scotland Coronary Prevention Study Group. *N Engl J Med* 1995;**333**:1301–1307.

107. Downs GR, Clearfield M, Weiss S *et al*. Primary prevention of acute coronary events with lovastatin in menand women with average cholesterol levels: results of AFCAPS/TEXCAPS. Air Force/Texas Coronary Atherosclerosis Study. *JAMA* 1998;**279**:1615–1622.

108. Heart Protection Study Collaborative Group. MRC/BHF Heart Protection Study of cholesterol lowering with simvastatin in 20 536 high-risk individuals: a randomized placebo-controlled trial. *Lancet* 2002;**360**:7–22.

109. Crouse JR, 3rd, ByingtonRP, Hoen HM, Furberg CD. Reductase inhibitor monotherapy and stroke prevention. *Arch Intern Med* 1997;**157**:1305–1310.

110. Herbert PR, Gaziano JM, Chan KS *et al*. Cholesterol lowering with statin drugs, risk of stroke, and total mortality. An overview of randomized trials. *JAMA* 1997;**278**:313–321.

111. EUROASPIRE Study Group. EUROASPIRE. A European Society of Cardiology survey of secondary prevention of coronary heart disease: Principal results. *Eur Heart J* 1997;**18**;1569–1582.

112. EUROASPIRE II Study Group. Lifestyle and risk factor management and use of drug therapies in coronary patients from 15 countries. Principal results from EUROASPIRE II. Euro Heart Survey Programme. *Eur Heart J* 2001;**22**:554–572.

113. EUROASPIRE I and II Group. Clinical reality of coronary prevention guidelines: a comparison of EUROASPIRE I and II in nine countries. *Lancet* 2001;**357**:995–1001.

Appendix 1 – Drugs

Drug	Trade name	Preparation	Strength	Dosages	Comments	Side effects
Antiplatelet drugs						
Acetylsalicylic acid	Aspirin	Tablet	75, 300 mg	75 mg/day	Contraindications: Active peptic ulceration Haemophilia and other bleeding disorders Breastfeeding Cautions: Asthma Uncontrolled hypertension Pregnancy	Gastrointestinal haemorrhage; bronchospasm
	Angettes 75	Tablet	75 mg			
	Caprin	Tablet	75, 300 mg			
	Nu-Seals Aspirin	Tablet	75, 300 mg			
Clopidogrel	Plavix	Tablet	75 mg	75 mg/day	Contraindications: Active bleeding Breastfeeding Cautions: Avoid for first few days after MI and for 7 days after ischaemic stroke Liver and renal impairment Pregnancy	Haemorrhage; gastrointestinal disorders; headache; dizziness; vertigo; rash; pruritus; hepatic and billiary disorders; neutropenia
Dipyridamole	Dipyridamole	Tablet	25, 100 mg	300–600 mg/day	Cautions: Rapidly worsening angina Aortic stenosis Recent MI Heart failure Hypotension	Gastrointestinal effects; dizziness; headache; myalgia; hypotension; rarely worsening symptoms of CHD; increased bleeding during and after surgery
	Persantin	Tablet	25, 100 mg			
	Persantin Retard	Capsule	200 mg			

Drug	Trade name	Preparation	Strength	Dosages	Comments	Side effects
Antiplatelet drugs						
Aspirin with dipiridamole	Asasantin Retard	Capsule	Aspirin 25 mg + Dipiridamole 200 mg	One capsule 2 times/day		
Ticlodipine hydrochloride	Ticlid	Tablet	250 mg	250 mg 2 times/day	Contraindications: Haemorrhagic diathesis Bleeding History of leucopenia, thrombocytopenia or agranulocytosis Cautions: Hepatic and renal impairement Monitor full blood count Pregnancy Breastfeeding	Bleeding; blood disorders; nausea; diarrhoea; liver disorders

Drug	Trade name	Preparation	Strength	Dosages	Comments	Side effects
Beta-blockers						
Acebutolol	Sectral	Capsule Tablet	100, 200 mg 400 mg	400–800 mg/day	Contraindications: Asthma Chronic obstructive heart disease Uncontrolled heart failure Marked bradycardia Hypotension Prinzmetal's angina Sick-sinus syndrome AV block II and III degree Cardiogenic shock Severe peripheral arterial disease Phaeochromocytoma Cautions: Pregnancy Breastfeeding AV block I degree Renal and liver impairment Diabetes Myasthenia gravis Avoid abrupt withdrawal	Bradycardia; heart failure; hypotension; conduction disorders; bronchospasm; peripheral vasoconstruction; gastrointestinal disturbances; fatigue; sleep disturbances; rare reports of rashes and dry eyes; exacerbation of psoriasis
Atenolol	Atenolol Tenormin 25 Tenormin LS Tenormin	Tablet Tablet Tablet Tablet	25, 50, 100 mg 25 mg 50 mg 100 mg	25–100 mg/day		
Betaxolole (AH)	Kerlone	Tablet	20 mg	20–40 mg/day		
Bisoprolol	Bisoprolol Fumarate Cardicor Emcor Emcor LS Monocor	Tablet Tablet Tablet Tablet Tablet	5, 10 mg 1.25, 2.5, 3.75, 5, 7.5, 10 mg 10 mg 5 mg 5, 10 mg	5–10 mg/day (max 20 mg/day)		

Drug	Trade name	Preparation	Strength	Dosages	Comments	Side effects
Beta-blockers						
Carvedilol	Eucardic	Tablet	3.125, 6.25, 12.5, 25 mg	12.5–25 mg/day (max 50 mg/day)	Contrandications: Asthma Chronic obstructive heart disease Uncontrolled heart failure Marked bradycardia Hypotension Prinzmetal's angina Sick-sinus syndrome AV block II and III degree Cardiogenic shock Severe peripheral arterial disease Phaeochromocytoma Cautions: Pregnancy Breastfeeding AV block I degree Renal and liver impairment Diabetes Myasthenia gravis Avoid abrupt withdrawal	Bradycardia; heart failure; hypotension; conduction disorders; bronchospasm; peripheral vasoconstruction; gastrointestinal disturbances; fatigue; sleep disturbances; rare reports of rashes and dry eyes; exacerbation of psoriasis
Celiprolol hydrochloride (AH)	Celiprolol	Tablet	200, 400 mg	200–400 mg		
	Celectol	Tablet	200, 400 mg			
Labetolol Hydrochloride	Labetolol Hydrochloride	Tablet	100, 200, 400 mg	100–200 mg 2 times/day		
	Trandate	Tablet	50, 100, 200, 400 mg			
Metoprolol Tartrate	Metoprolol Tartrate	Tablet	50, 100 mg	100–300 mg/day		
	Betaloc	Tablet	50, 100 mg			
	Betaloc-SA	M/R tablet	200 mg			
	Lopressor	Tablet	50, 100 mg			
	Lopressor SR	M/R tablet	200 mg			

Drug	Trade name	Preparation	Strength	Dosages	Comments	Side effects
Beta-blockers						
Nadolol	Corgard	Tablet	40, 80 mg	80 mg/day (max 160 mg/day)	Contrandications: Asthma Chronic obstructive heart disease Uncontrolled heart failure Marked bradycardia Hypotension Prinzmetal's angina Sick-sinus syndrome AV block II and III degree Cardiogenic shock Severe peripheral arterial disease Phaeochromocytoma Cautions: Pregnancy Breastfeeding AV block I degree Renal and liver impairment Diabetes Myasthenia gravis Avoid abrupt withdrawal	Bradycardia; heart failure; hypotension; conduction disorders; bronchospasm; peripheral vasoconstruction; gastrointestinal disturbances; fatigue; sleep disturbances; rare reports of rashes and dry eyes; exacerbation of psoriasis
Nebivolol (AH)	Nelibet	Tablet	5 mg	5 mg/day		
Oxprenolol hydrochloride	Oxprenolol	Tablet	20, 40, 80, 160 mg	80–160 mg/day (max 320 mg)		
	Trasicor	Tablet	20, 40, 80 mg			
	Slow-Trasicor	Tablet	160 mg			
Pindolol	Visken	Tablet	5, 15 mg	2,5–5mg 2–3 times/day (max 45 mg/day)		

Drug	Trade name	Preparation	Strength	Dosages	Comments	Side effects
Beta-blockers						
Propranolol hydrochloride	Propranolol	Tablet	10, 40, 80, 160 mg	80–240 mg/day	Contrandications: Asthma Chronic obstructive heart disease Uncontrolled heart failure Marked bradycardia Hypotension Prinzmetal's angina Sick-sinus syndrome AV block II and III degree Cardiogenic shock Severe peripheral arterial disease Phaeochromocytoma Cautions: Pregnancy Breastfeeding AV block I degree Renal and liver impairment Diabetes Myasthenia gravis Avoid abrupt withdrawal	Bradycardia; heart failure; hypotension; conduction disorders; bronchospasm; peripheral vasoconstruction; gastrointestinal disturbances; fatigue; sleep disturbances; rare reports of rashes and dry eyes; exacerbation of psoriasis
	Inderal	Tablet	10, 40, 80 mg			
	Half-Inderal LA	M/R Capsule	80 mg			
	Inderal-LA	M/R Capsule	160 mg			
Sotalol hydrochloride (arrhythmias)						
Timolol Maleate	Betim	Tablet	10 mg	15– 45 mg/day (max 60 mg/day)		

Drug	Trade name	Preparation	Strength	Dosages	Comments	Side effects
Angiotensin-converting enzyme inhibitors						
Captopril	Captopril	Tablet	12.5, 25, 50 mg	Initially 6.25 mg (max 150 mg/day)	Contraindications: Renovascular disease Aortic stenosis Outflow tract obstruction Cautions: Renal and hepatic impairment Pregnancy Breastfeeding Initiate treatment with low doses	Hypotension; renal impairment; persistent dry cough; angioedema; rash; pancreatitis; upper respiratory tract symptoms; gastrointestinal effects; liver function alteration; blood disorders; headache, dizziness; fatigue; malaise; taste disturbances; myalgia; photosensitivity
	Capoten	Tablet	12.5, 25, 50 mg	Initially 6.25 mg (max 150 mg/day)		
Cilazapril (AH, HF)	Vascace	Tablet	0.5, 1, 2.5 mg	1–2.5 mg/day (max 5 mg/day)		
Enalapril maleate	Enalapril Maleate	Tablet	2.5, 5, 10, 20 mg	5–40 mg/day		
	Innovace	Tablet	2.5, 5, 10, 20 mg	5–40 mg/day		
Fosinopril (AH, HF)	Staril	Tablet	10, 20 mg	10–40 mg/day		
Imidapril hydrochloride (AH)	Tanatril	Tablet	5, 10, 20 mg	5–20 mg/day		

Drug	Trade name	Preparation	Strength	Dosages	Comments	Side effects
Angiotensin-converting enzyme inhibitors						
Imidapril hydrochloride (AH)	Tanatril	Tablet	5, 10, 20 mg	5–20 mg/day	Contraindications: Renovascular disease Aortic stenosis Outflow tract obstruction Cautions: Renal and hepatic impairment Pregnancy Breastfeeding Initiate treatment with low doses	Hypotension; renal impairment; persistent dry cough; angioedema; rash; pancreatitis; upper respiratory tract symptoms; gastrointestinal effects; liver function alteration; blood disorders; headache, dizziness; fatigue; malaise; taste disturbances; myalgia; photosensitivity
Lisinopril	Carace	Tablet	2.5, 5, 10, 20 mg	2.5–10 mg/day		
	Zestril	Tablet	2.5, 5, 10, 20 mg	2.5–10 mg/day		
Moexipril hydrochloryde (AH)	Perdix	Tablet	7.5, 15 mg	7.5–30 mg/day		
Perindopril (AH, HF)	Coversyl	Tablet	2, 4 mg	2–4 mg/day (max 8 mg/day)		
Quinapril (AH, HF)	Accupro	Tablet	5, 10, 20, 40 mg	5–40 mg/day		
Ramipril	Tritace	Tablet	1.25, 2.5, 5, 10 mg	5–10 mg/day		
Trandolapril	Gopten	Capsule	0.5, 1, 2 mg	0.5–4 mg/day		
	Odrik	Capsule	0.5, 1, 2 mg	0.5–4 mg/day		

Drug	Trade name	Preparation	Strength	Dosages	Comments	Side effects
Angiotensin-II receptor antagonists						
Candesartan Cilexetil (AH)	Amias	Tablet	2, 4, 8, 16 mg	4–8 mg/day (max 16 mg/day)	Contraindications: Pregnancy Breastfeeding Billiary obstruction (telmisartan and valsartan) Cautions: Aortic valve stenosis Mitral valve stenosis Obstructive hypertrophic cardiomyopathy Renal impairment Hepatic impairment	Symptomatic hypotension; hyperkalaemia; angioedema; reported gastrointestinal disturbances (diarrhoea, dyspepsia); arthralgia; myalgia; dizziness; headache; rush; urticaria; rhinitis; pharyngitis; blood disorders; fatigue
Eprosartan (AH)	Teveten	Tablet	300, 400, 600 mg	300–800 mg/day		
Irbesartan (AH)	Aprovel	Tablet	75, 150, 300 mg	150–300 mg/day		
Losartan Potassium (AH)	Cozaar	Tablet	25, 50, 100 mg	50–100 mg/day		
Telmisartan	Micardis	Tablet	20, 40, 80 mg	40–80 mg/day		
Valsartan	Diovan	Capsule	40, 80, 160 mg	80–160 mg/day		

Drug	Trade name	Preparation	Strength	Dosages	Comments	Side effects
Calcium-channel blockers						
Amlodipine Besilate	Istin	Tablet	5,10 mg	5 mg/day (max 10 mg/day)	Contraindications: Cardiogenic shock Unstable angina Aortic stenosis Pregnancy Breastfeeding Caution: Renal impairment Hepatic impairment	Headache; oedema; fatigue; nausea; flushing; dizziness; rarely gastrointestinal disturbances; dry mouth; sweating; palpitations; dyspnoea; drowsiness; mood changes; myalgia; arthralgia; asthenia; peripheral neuropathy; impotence; increased urinary frequency; visual disturbances; gynaecomastia
Diltiazem hydrochloride	Diltiazem	Tablets	60 mg	60 mg 3 times/day (max 360 mg/day)	Contraindications: Severe bradycardia Left ventricular failure Second or third degree AV block Sick-sinus syndrome Pregnancy Breastfeeding Caution: Renal failure Bradycardia First-degree AV block	Bradycardia; sino-atrial block; AV block; palpitations; dizziness; hypotension; headache; hot flushes; gastrointestinal disturbances; oedema; rashes; hepatitis; gynaecomastia
	Adizem-SR	M/R capsule	90,120 180 mg	120 mg 2 times/day (max 180 mg 2 times/day		

Drug	Trade name	Preparation	Strength	Dosages	Comments	Side effects
Calcium-channel blockers						
Diltiazem hydrochloride	Adizem-XL	M/R capsule	120, 180, 240, 300 mg	240 mg/day (120 mg/day elderly, renal and hepatic impairment)	Contraindications: Severe bradycardia Left ventricular failure Second or third degree AV block Sick-sinus syndrome Pregnancy Breastfeeding Caution: Renal failure Bradycardia First-degree AV block	Bradycardia; sino-atrial block; AV block; palpitations; dizziness; hypotension; headache; hot flushes; gastrointestinal disturbances; oedema; rashes; hepatitis; gynaecomastia
	Angitil SR	M/R capsule	90, 180 mg	90 mg 2 times/day (max 180 mg two times/day)		
	Angitil XL	M/R capsule	240, 300 mg	240 mg/day (max 360 mg/day)		
	Calcicard CR	M/R capsule	90, 120 mg	90–120 mg 2 times/day (max 360 mg/day)		
	Dilcardia SR	M/R capsule	60, 90, 120 mg	90–120 mg 2 times/day (max 360 mg/day)		

Drug	Trade name	Preparation	Strength	Dosages	Comments	Side effects
Calcium-channel blockers						
Diltiazem Hydrochloride	Dilzem SR	M/R capsule	60, 90, 120 mg	90–120 mg 2 times/day (max 360 mg/day)	Contraindications: Severe bradycardia Left ventricular failure Second or third degree AV block Sick-sinus syndrome Pregnancy Breastfeeding Caution: Renal failure Bradycardia First-degree AV block	Bradycardia; sino-atrial block; AV block; palpitations; dizziness; hypotension; headache; hot flushes; gastrointestinal disturbances; oedema; rashes; hepatitis; gynaecomastia
	Dilzem XL	M/R capsule	120, 180, 240 mg	180 mg/day (max 360 mg/day)		
	Slozem	M/R capsule	120, 180, 240, 300 mg	240 mg/day (max 360 mg/day)		
	Tildiem	M/R Tablets	60 mg	60 mg 3 times/day (max 360 mg/day)		
	Tildiem LA	M/R capsule	200, 300 mg	200 mg/day, increased to 300–400 mg/day (max 500 mg/day, 300 mg/day elderly, renal and hepatic impairment)		

Drug	Trade name	Preparation	Strength	Dosages	Comments	Side effects
Calcium-channel blockers						
Diltiazem hydrochloride	Tildiem Retard	M/R tablets	90, 120 mg	90–120 mg 2 times/day, 120 mg/day elderly, renal and hepatic impairment (max 360 mg/day)	Contraindications: Severe bradycardia Left ventricular failure Second or third-degree AV block Sick-sinus syndrome Pregnancy Breastfeeding Caution: Renal failure Bradycardia First-degree AV block	Bradycardia; sino-atrial block; AV block; palpitations; dizziness; hypotension; headache; hot flushes; gastrointestinal disturbances; oedema; rashes; hepatitis; gynaecomastia
	Viazem XL	M/R capsule	120, 180, 240, 300, 360 mg	120–300 (360) mg/day		
	Zemtard	Capsules	120, 180, 240, 300 XL	120–300 (360) mg/day		
Felodipine	Plendil	Tablets	2.5, 5, 10 mg	5–10 mg/day	Contraindications: Unstable angina Significant aortic stenosis Pregnancy Uncontrolled heart failure Within 1 month of MI Caution: Renal impairment Hepatic impairment Breastfeeding	Palpitations; dizziness; hypotension; headache; flushing; fatigue; gravitational oedema; rashes

Drug	Trade name	Preparation	Strength	Dosages	Comments	Side effects
Calcium-channel blockers						
Isradipine (AH)	Prescal	Tablets	2.5 mg	2.5–5 mg/day (max 10 mg 2 times/day)	Contraindications: Tight aortic stenosis Sick-sinus syndrome Pregnancy Caution: Renal impairment Hepatic impairment	Tachycardia; palpitations; dizziness; headache; flushing; fatigue; rashes
Lacidipine (AH)	Motens	Tablets	2, 4 mg	2–4 mg/day (max 6 mg/day)	Contraindications: Aortic stenosis Pregnancy Breastfeeding Within 1 month of MI Caution: Renal impairment Hepatic impairment	Palpitations; dizziness; hypotension; headache; flushing; fatigue; oedema; rashes

Drug	Trade name	Preparation	Strength	Dosages	Comments	Side effects
Calcium-channel blockers						
Lercanidipine hydrochloride (AH)	Zanidip	Tablet	10 mg		Contraindications: Unstable angina Aortic stenosis Uncontrolled heart failure Pregnancy Breastfeeding Within 1 month of MI Caution: Renal impairment Hepatic impairment Left ventricular dysfunction Sick-sinus syndrome	Tachycarida; palpitations; dizziness; hypotension; headache; flushing; fatigue; rashes; peripheral oedema; asthenia
Nicardipine hydrochloride	Nicardipine	Capsules	20,30 mg	20 mg 3 times/day, usual range 60–120 mg/day	Contraindications: Cardiogenic shock Unstable angina Aortic stenosis Pregnancy Breastfeeding Within 1 month of MI Caution: Congestive heart failure Significantly impaired left ventricular function Renal impairment Hepatic impairment	Palpitations; dizziness; hypotension; headache; flushing; fatigue; rashes; peripheral oedema; asthenia; gastrointestinal disturbances
	Cardene	Capsules	20,30 mg	20 mg 3 times/day, usual range 60–120 mg/day		
	Cardene SR	M/R capsule	30, 45 mg	30 mg 2 times/day, usual range 30–60 mg		

Drug	Trade name	Preparation	Strength	Dosages	Comments	Side effects
Calcium-channel blockers						
Nifedipine	Nifedipine	Capsules	5, 10mg	Not recommended	Contraindications: Cardiogenic shock Unstable angina Aortic stenosis Pregnancy Breastfeeding Within 1 month of MI Caution: Congestive heart failure Significantly impaired left ventricular function Renal impairment Hepatic impairment	Palpitations; dizziness; hypotension; headache; flushing; fatigue; rashes; peripheral oedema; asthenia; gastrointestinal disturbances
	Adalat	Capsules	5, 10mg	Not recommended		
	Adalat LA	M/R tablets	20, 30, 60 mg	30 mg/day (max 90 mg/day)		
	Adalat Retard	M/R tablets	10, 20 mg	10 mg 2 times/day (max 40 mg 2 times/day)		
	Adipine MR	M/R tablets	10, 20 mg	10 mg 2 times/day (max 40 mg 2 times/day)		
	Cardilate MR	M/R tablets	10, 20 mg	20 mg 2 times/day (max 80 mg/day)		
	Coracten SR	M/R tablets	10, 20 mg	20 mg 2 times/day (max 80 mg/day)		

Drug	Trade name	Preparation	Strength	Dosages	Comments	Side effects
Calcium-channel blockers						
Nisoldipine	Syscor MR	M/R tablets	10, 20, 30 mg	10–20 mg/day (max 40 mg/day)	Contraindications: Cardiogenic shock Unstable angina Aortic stenosis Pregnancy Breastfeeding Within 1 month of MI Hepatic impairment Caution: Renal impairment	Palpitations; tachycardia; dizziness; nausea; hypotension; headache; flushing; fatigue; rashes; gravitational oedema; asthenia; gastrointestinal disturbances
Verapamil hydro-chloride	Verapamil	Tablets	40, 80, 120, 160 mg	80–120 mg 3 times/ day	Contraindications: Bradycardia Cardiogenic shock Hypotension Left ventricular failure Second or third-degree AV block Sick-sinus syndrome Porphyria Atrial flutter or fibrillation complicated WPW syndrome Caution: First-degree AV block Acute phase of MI Hepatic impairment Pregnancy Breastfeeding	Constipation; dizziness; nausea; hypotension; headache; flushing; ankle oedema; bradycardia; heart block; allergic reactions
	Cordilox	Tablets	40, 80, 120, 160 mg	80–120 mg 3 times /day		
	Securon	Tablets	40, 120 mg	120 (240) mg/day		
	Half Securon SR	M/R tablets	120 mg	240 (360) mg/day		
	Securon SR	M/R tablets	240 mg	240 (360) mg/day		
	Univer	M/R capsule	120, 180, 240 mg	240 (360) mg/day		
	Verapress MR	M/R tablets	240 mg	240 mg/day		
	Vertab SR 240	M/R tablets	240 mg	240 mg/day		

Drug	Trade name	Preparation	Strength	Dosages	Comments	Side effects
Lipid-lowering drugs						
Anion-exchange resins						
Colestyramine	Colestyramine Questran Questran Light	Sachet Sachet Sachet	4 mg 4 mg 4 mg	12–24 g/day in water or up to four divided doses/day. Initiate treatment with low doses, and use low doses, e.g. 4–8 g at bedtime, when colestyramine is used in combination with statins	For treatment of primary hypercholesterolaemia Contraindications: Complete biliary obstruction Hypertriglyceridaemia Pregnancy Breastfeeding Cautions: Anion-exchange resins interfere with the absorption of fat-soluble vitamins; supplements of vitamins A, D and K may be required when treatment is prolonged Decrease the absorption of other drugs Initiate treatment with low doses and use low doses at bedtime, when resin is used in combination with statins	Gastrointestinal effects; increased bleeding associated with vitamin K deficiency
Colestipol hydrochloride	Colestid	Sachet	5 g	5–10 g /day in liquid increased if necessary to max of 30 g/day		

Drug	Trade name	Preparation	Strength	Dosages	Comments	Side effects
Lipid-lowering drugs						
Cholesterol-absorption inhibitor						
Ezetimibe	Ezetrol (Germany)	Tablet	10 mg	10 mg/day	For treatment of primary hypercholesterolaemia as an adjuvant to statin therapy Contraindications: Hepatic insufficiency Pregnancy Breastfeeding	
	Zetia (USA)	Tablet	10 mg	10 mg/day		
Fibrates						
Bezafibrate	Bezafibrate	Tablet	200 mg	200 mg 3 times/day after food	For treatment of mixed dyslipidaemias Contraindications: Severe hepatic or renal insufficiency Primary biliary cirrhosis Gallbladder disease Pregnancy Breastfeeding Cautions: Renal impairment (reduce dose) Combination with statins	Gastrointestinal effects; pruritus; urticaria; headache; dizziness; vertigo; fatigue; hair loss; myotoxicity (increased risk of rhabdomyolysis in patients with renal impairment and in combination with a statin
	Bezalip	Tablet	200 mg	200 mg 3 times/ day with or after food		
	Bezalip Mono	M/R tablet	400 mg	400 mg/day after food		
Ciprofibrate	Modalim	Tablet	100 mg	100 mg/day		

Drug	Trade name	Preparation	Strength	Dosages	Comments	Side effects
Lipid-lowering drugs						
Fibrates						
Fenofibrate	Lipantil Micro 67	Capsule	67 mg	Three capsules/ day after food; usual range two–four capsules/day	For treatment of mixed dyslipidaemias Contraindications: Severe hepatic or renal insufficiency Primary biliary cirrhosis Gallbladder disease Pregnancy Breastfeeding Cautions: Renal impairment (reduce dose) Combination with statins	Gastrointestinal effects; pruritus; urticaria; headache; dizziness; vertigo; fatigue; hair loss; myotoxicity (increased risk of rhabdomyolysis in patients with renal impairment and in combination with a statin
	Lipantil Micro 200	Capsule	200 mg	One capsule/day after food		
	Lipantil Micro 267	Capsule	267 mg	One capsule /day		
	Supralip 160	M/R tablet	160 mg	160 mg/day		
Gemfibrozil	Gemfibrozil	Capsule	300 mg	600 mg 2 times/day (range 0.9–1.5g/ day)		
		Tablet	600 mg			
	Lopid	Capsule	300 mg	600 mg 2 times/day (range 0.9–1.5g/ day)		
		Tablet	600 mg			

Drug	Trade name	Preparation	Strength	Dosages	Comments	Side effects
Lipid-lowering drugs						
Statins						
Atorvastatin	Lipitor	Tablet	10, 20, 40, 80 mg	10–40 mg/day (max 80 mg/day)	For treatment of primary hyper-cholesterolaemia, including familial hyper-cholesterolaemia, and mixed dyslipidaemias Contraindications: Active liver disease Pregnancy Breastfeeding Cautions: History of liver disease (liver function tests should be carried out before and within 1–3 months of starting and thereafter at intervals of 6 months. Treatment should be discontinued if serum transaminase concentration rises to three times the upper limit.) In combination with fibrate, nicotinic acid, immunosuppressants (ciclosporin) Patient should be advised to report unexplained muscle pain. If the creatine kinase concentration is elevated (> 10 times upper limit), and myopathy is suspected or diagnosed, treatment should be discontinued.	Muscle effects: myalgia, myositis and myopathy; increased incidence of myopathy and rhabdomyolysis if the statins are given with a fibrate; altered liver function; headache; gastrointestinal effects; rash
	Zarator	Tablet	10, 20, 40, 80 mg			
Fluvastatin	Lescol	Capsule	20, 40 mg	20–40 mg in the evening (max 80 mg/day)		
	Lescol XL	M/R tablets	80 mg	80 mg/day		
	Canef	Capsule	20,40 mg			
Lovastatin	Mevacor	Tablet	20,40 mg	20, 40 mg evening (max 80 mg)		
Pravastatin sodium	Lipostat	Tablet	10, 20, 40 mg	10–40 mg/day in the evening		
	Pravachol	Tablet	10, 20, 40 mg			
Rosuvastatin	Crestor	Tablet	10, 20, 40 mg	10–20 mg/ any time of day (max 40 mg/day)		
Simvastatin	Zocor	Tablet	10, 20, 40, 80 mg	10–40 mg/day in the evening (max 80 mg/day)		

<table>
<tr><th>Drug</th><th>Trade name</th><th>Preparation</th><th>Strength</th><th>Dosages</th><th>Comments</th><th>Side effects</th></tr>
<tr><td colspan="7">Lipid-lowering drugs</td></tr>
<tr><td colspan="7">Nicotinic acid group</td></tr>
<tr><td>Acipimox</td><td>Olbetam</td><td>Capsule</td><td>250 mg</td><td>500–750 mg/day in divided doses</td><td rowspan="2">For treatment of dyslipidaemias including mixed dyslipidaemias and hypercholesterolaemia. In doses 1.5–3 g/day it lowers both cholesterol and triglycerides, and increases HDL-cholesterol

Contraindications:
Pregnancy
Breastfeeding
Chronic liver disease
Peptic ulcer
Severe gout

Cautions:
Diabetes mellitus
Hyperuricaemia</td><td rowspan="2">Vasodilatation; flushing; itching; rashes; urticaria; erythema; gastrointestinal effects; headache; impaired liver function</td></tr>
<tr><td>Nicotinic acid</td><td>Nicotinic acid</td><td>Tablet</td><td>50 mg</td><td>100–200 mg 3 times/day increased over 2-4 weeks to 1–2 g 3 times/day</td></tr>
</table>

Drug	Trade name	Preparation	Strength	Dosages	Comments	Side effects
Lipid-lowering drugs						
Fish oils						
Omega-3-acid ethyl esters	Omacor	Capsules	1 g of 90% omega-3 acid ethyl esters containing eicosapentaenoic acid 46% and docosahexaenoic acid 38%, alpha-tocopherol 4 mg	One capsule/day with food	For treatment of hypertriglyceridaemia and secondary prevention of cardiovascular disease Cautions: Haemorrhagic disorders Anticoagulant treatment	Nausea; belching; diarrhoea; constipation; eczema; acne
Omega-3-marine triglycerides	MaxEPA	Capsules Liquid	1 g (approx 1.1 ml) of fish oil containing eicosapentaenoic acid 170 mg, docosahexaenoic acid 115 mg, vitamin A (< 100 units/g) and vitamin D (< 10 units/g)	Five capsules 2 times/day with food	For treatment of hypertriglyceridaemia and secondary prevention of cardiovascular disease Cautions: Haemorrhagic disorders Anticoagulant treatment Aspirin-sensitive asthma Diabetes mellitus	Nausea; belching

Drug	Trade name	Preparation	Strength	Dosages	Comments	Side effects
Oral anticoagulants						
Warfarin sodium	Warfarin	Tablet	0.5, 1, 3, 5 mg	10 mg/day for 2 days, then depending on the prothrombin time, reported as INT. Maintenance dose 3–9 mg (taken at the same time each day)	Contraindications: Pregnancy Peptic ulcer Severe hypertension Bacterial endocarditis Cautions: Hepatic and renal disease Breastfeeding	Haemorrhage; rash; alopecia; gastrointestinal effects; hepatic dysfunction
Aceno-coumarol/ Nicoumalone	Sinthrome	Tablet	1 mg	8–12 mg 1st day, 4–8 mg 2nd day, maintenance dose 1–8 mg/day (see Warfarin sodium)	*See* Warfarin sodium	*See* Warfarin sodium
Phenindione	Phenindione	Tablet	10, 25, 50 mg	200 mg 1st day, 100 mg 2nd day, maintenance dose 50–150 mg/day	*See* Warfarin sodium	*See* Warfarin sodium

Drug	Trade name	Preparation	Strength	Dosages	Comments	Side effects
Nicotine-replacement therapy						
Nicorette	Nicorette Microtab	Sublingual tablet	2 mg	2–4 mg each hour (max 80 mg/day) for at least 3 months followed by a gradual reduction in dosage (max 6 months)	Contraindications: Severe cardiovascular disease Recent cerebrovascular incident Pregnancy Breastfeeding Patches, chronic generalised skin disease Child under 18 years not recommended Cautions: Cardiovascular disease Hyperthyroidism Diabetes mellitus Phaeochromocytoma Renal and hepatic impairment History of gastritis and peptic ulcer Should not smoke in combination with nicotine replacement therapy	Nausea; dizziness; headache; cold and influenza-like symptoms; palpitations; gastrointestinal effects; insomnia; myalgia; blood pressure changes
	Nicorette chewing gum	Chewing gum	2, 4 mg	2–4 mg chewed for approx. 30 min when urge to smoke; withdraw gradually after 3 months		
	Nicorette patches	Patches	5, 10, 15 mg	15-mg patch for 16 hours/day for 8 weeks, then 10-mg patch for 2 weeks, then 5-mg patch for 2 weeks		
	Nicorette nasal spray	Nasal spray	500 μg/metered spray	One spray into each nostril to max twice/hr		

Drug	Trade name	Preparation	Strength	Dosages	Comments	Side effects
Nicotine-replacement therapy						
Nicorette	Nicorette inhalator	Inhalator	10 mg/cartridge	Inhale when urge to smoke, six–12 cartridges/day for up to 8 weeks, then reduce number of cartridges by half over next 2 weeks	Contraindications: Severe cardiovascular disease Recent cerebrovascular incident Pregnancy Breastfeeding Patches, chronic generalised skin disease Child under 18 years not recommended Cautions: Cardiovascular disease Hyperthyroidism Diabetes mellitus Phaeochromocytoma Renal and hepatic impairment History of gastritis and peptic ulcer Should not smoke in combination with nicotine replacement therapy	Nausea; dizziness; headache; cold and influenza-like symptoms; palpitations; gastrointestinal effects; insomnia; myalgia; blood pressure changes
Nicotinell	Nicotinell chewing gum	Chewing gum	2, 4 mg	2 mg chewed for approx. 30 min when urge to smoke; max 15 pieces/day		
	Nicotinell mint lozenge	Mint lozenge	1 mg	One lozenge every 1–2 hours when urge to smoke; max 25 lozenges/day; withdraw gradually after 3 months		
	Nicotinell TTS Patches	Patches "10" patch "20" patch "30" patch	 7 mg 14 mg 21 mg	"20" to "30" patch/day reducing dose every 3–4 weeks		

Drug	Trade name	Preparation	Strength	Dosages	Comments	Side effects
Nicotine-replacement therapy						
NiQuitin CQ	NiQuitin CQ lozenges	Lozenges	2, 4 mg	One lozenge every 1–2 hr when urge to smoke; max 15 lozenges/day; withdraw gradually after 3 months	Contraindications: Severe cardiovascular disease Recent cerebrovascular incident Pregnancy Breastfeeding Patches, chronic generalised skin disease Child under 18 years not recommended Cautions: Cardiovascular disease Hyperthyroidism Diabetes mellitus Phaeochromocytoma Renal and hepatic impairment History of gastritis and peptic ulcer Should not smoke in combination with nicotine replacement therapy	Nausea; dizziness; headache; cold and influenza-like symptoms; palpitations; gastrointestinal effects; insomnia; myalgia; blood pressure changes
	NiQuitin CQ patches	Patches	7, 14, 21 mg	Initially "21-mg" patch/day for 6 weeks, then "14-mg" patch/day for 2 weeks then "7-mg" patch/day for 2 weeks		
Bupropion (Amfe-butamone)	Zyban	M/R tablet	150 mg	Initially 150 mg/day for 6 days, then 150 mg 2 times/day; max period of treatment 7–9 weeks	Contraindications: History of seizures Eating disorders and bipolar disorder Pregnancy Breastfeeding Cautions: Elderly people Hepatic or renal impairment Predisposition to seizures	Gastrointestinal effects; insomnia; tremor; impaired concentration; headache; dizziness; depression; anxiety; rush; pruritus; sweating

Drug	Trade name	Preparation	Strength	Dosages	Comments	Side effects
Anti-obesity agents						
Orlistat	Xenical	Capsule	120 mg	120 mg up to 3 times/ day immediately before, during or up to 1 hr after each main meal	Contraindications: Chronic malabsorption syndrome Cholestasis Pregnancy Breastfeeding Cautions: Diabetes mellitus	Liquid oily stools; faecal urgency; flatulence; abdominal and rectal pain; headache; menstrual irregularities; anxiety; fatigue; rarely hepatitis
Sibutramine hydrochloride	Reductil	Capsule	10, 15 mg	10–15mg/ day in the morning	Contraindications: Major eating disorders Psychiatric illness Tourette's syndrome History of CHD, congestive heart failure, tachycardia, arrhythmias, peripheral arterial occlusive disease, cerebrovascular disease Uncontrolled hypertension Hyperthyroidism Phaeochromocytoma Prostatic hypertrophy Pregnancy Breastfeeding Cautions: Monitor blood pressure and heart rate Sleep apnoea syndrome Epilepsy Hepatic impairment Renal impairment	Constipation; anorexia; dry mouth; insomnia; nausea; tachycardia; palpitations; hypertension; vasodilatation; paraesthesia; headache; anxiety; sweating; taste disturbance; rarely blurred vision

Appendix 2 – Cardiovascular prevention guidelines

Europe

Pyörälä K, De Backer G, Graham I *et al*. Prevention of coronary heart disease in clinical practice. Recommendations of the Task Force of the European Society of Cardiology, European Atherosclerotic Society and European Society of Hypertension. *Eur Heart J* 1994;**15**:1300–1331.

Wood D, De Backer G, Faergeman O *et al*. Prevention of coronary heart disease in clinical practice. Recommendations of the Second Joint Task Force of European and Other Societies on Coronary Prevention. *Eur Heart J* 1998;**19**:1434–1503.

De Backer G, Ambrosioni E, Borch-Johnsen K *et al*. European guidelines on cardiovascular disease prevention in clinical practice. Executive Summary. Third Joint Task Force of European and Other Societies on Cardiovascular Disease Prevention in Clinical Practice (constituted by representatives of eight societies and by invited experts). *Eur J Cardiovasc Prev Rehabil* 2003;**10**:S1–S10; *Eur Heart J* 2003;**24**:1601–1610.

De Backer G, Ambrosioni E, Borch-Johnsen K *et al*. European guidelines on cardiovascular disease prevention in clinical practice. Third Joint Task Force of European and Other Societies on Cardiovascular Disease Prevention in Clinical Practice (constituted by representatives of eight societies and by invited experts). *Eur J Cardiovasc Rehabil* 2003;**10** (Suppl. 1):S1–S78.

UK

Joint British recommendations on prevention of coronary heart disease in clinical practice: summary. British Cardiac Society, British Hyperlipidaemia Association, British Hypertension Society, British Diabetic Association. *BMJ* 2000;**320**:705–708.

Wood DA, Durrington P, Poulter N *et al*. on behalf of the British Cardiac Society, British Hyperlipidaemia Association, British Hypertension Society, British Diabetic Association. Joint British recommendations on prevention of coronary heart disease in clinical practice. *Heart* 1998;**80**(Suppl. 2): S1–S29.

Ramsay LE, Williams B, Johnston GD *et al*. British Hypertension Society guidelines for hypertension management 1999: summary. *BMJ* 1999;**319**:630–635.

Ramsay L, Williams B, Johnston G *et al*. Guidelines for management of hypertension: report of the Third working party of the British Hypertension Society. *J Hum Hypertens* 1999;**13**:569–592.

USA

National Institutes of Health. Third Report of the National Cholesterol Education Program (NCEP) Expert Panel on Detection, Evaluation, and Treatment of High Blood Cholesterol in Adults (Adult Treatment Panel III). Executive Summary. NIH Publication No 01-3670. Bethesda: National Institues of Health, May 2001.

The Seventh Report of the Joint National Committee on Prevention, Detection, Evaluation, and Treatment of High Blood Pressure. The JNC 7 Report. *JAMA* 2003;**289**:2560–2572.

Expert Committee on the Diagnosis and Classification of Diabetes Mellitus. Report of the expert committee on the diagnosis and classification of diabetes mellitus. American Diabetes Association: Clinical Practice Recommendations 2001: Committee report. *Diabetes Care* 2002;**25**:S5–S20.

Appendix 3 – Lifestyle risk factor and therapeutic goals

	Europe	UK	USA
Patients with established atherosclerotic disease			
Lifestyle	- No smoking - Make healthy food choices - Be physically active	- No smoking - Make healthy food choices - Be physically active	- No smoking - Make healthy food choices - Be physically active
Body mass index	< 25 kg/m^2	< 25 kg/m^2	< 25 kg/m^2
Waist circumference	< 102 cm in men < 88 cm in women	< 102 cm in men < 88 cm in women	< 102 cm in men < 88 cm in women
Blood pressure	< 140/90 mmHg in most < 130/80 mmHg in particular groups	< 140/85 mmHg	< 140/90 mmHg < 130/80 mmHg (for patients with diabetes or chronic kidney disease)
Total cholesterol	< 4.5 mmol/l (175 mg/dl)	< 5 mmol/l	
LDL cholesterol	< 2.5 mmol/l (100 mg/dl)	< 3 mmol/l	< 2.5 mmol/l (100 mg/dl)
Diabetes *Type 1 diabetes*: HbA1c Fasting glucose Postprandial glucose	Optimal glucose control 6.2–7.5% 5.1–6.5 mmol/l (91–120 mg/dl) 7.6–9.0 mmol/l (136–160 mg/dl)	Optimal glucose control	Optimal glucose control

	Europe	UK	USA
Patients with established atherosclerotic disease			
Type 2 diabetes: HBA1c (DCCT-standardized)	≤ 6.1%	< 7.5% or < 6.5%*	≤ 7%
Venous plasma glucose:			
Fasting/preprandial	≤ 6.0 mmol/l (< 110 mg/dl)		5.0–7.2 mmol/l (90–130 mg/dl)
Peak postprandial			< 10 mmol/l (180 mg/dl)
Self-monitored blood glucose:			
Fasting/preprandial	4.0–5.0 mmol/l (70–90 mg/dl)		
Postprandial	4.0–7.5 mmol/l (70–135 mg/dl)		
Blood pressure	< 130/80 mmHg	< 130/80 mmHg (<125/75 when there is proteinuria)	< 130/80 mmHg
Total cholesterol	< 4.5 mmol/l (175 mg/dl)	< 5.0 mmol/l	
LDL-cholesterol	< 2.5 mmol/l (100 mg/dl)	< 3.0 mmol/l	< 2.6 mmol/l (100 mg/dl)
HDL-cholesterol			> 1.1 mmol/l (40 mg/dl)
Triglycerides			< 1.7 mmol/l (150 mg/dl)

* For patients at significant risk of macrovascular complications

	Europe	UK	USA
Asymptomatic subjects at high multifactorial risk			
Lifestyle	- No smoking - Make healthy food choices - Be physically active	- No smoking - Make healthy food choices - Be physically active	- No smoking - Make healthy food choices - Be physically active
Body mass index	< 25 kg/m^2	< 25 kg/m^2	< 25 kg/m^2
Waist circumference	< 102 cm in men < 88 cm in women	< 102 cm in men < 88 cm in women	< 102 cm in men < 88 cm in women
Blood pressure	< 140/90 mmHg in most < 130/80 mmHg in particular groups	< 140/85 mmHg	< 140/90 mmHg < 130/80 mmHg (for patients with diabetes or chronic kidney disease)
Total cholesterol	< 4.5 mmol/l (175 mg/dl) for patients whose untreated value is close to 5.0 mmol/l < 5.0 mmol/l(190 mg/dl) for patients with higher untreated values	< 5 mmol/l)	
LDL-cholesterol	< 2.5 mmol/l (100 mg/dl) for patients whose untreated value is close to 3.0 mmol/l < 3.0 mmol/l (115 mg/dl) for patients with higher untreated values	< 3 mmol/l	< 3.25 mmol/l (130 mg/dl) (for people with multiple (2+) risk factors)

	Europe	UK	USA
Asymptomatic subjects at high multifactorial risk			
Diabetes	Optimal glucose control	Optimal glucose control	Optimal glucose control
Type 1 diabetes:			
HbA1c	6.0–7.5%		
Fasting glucose	5.1–6.5 mmol/l (91–120 mg/dl)		
Postprandial glucose	7.6–9.0 mmol/l (136–160 mg/dl)		
Type 2 diabetes:			
HBA1c (DCCT standardized)	≤ 6.1%	< 7.5% or < 6.5%*	≤ 7%
Venous plasma glucose			
Fasting/preprandial	≤ 6.0 mmol/l (< 110 mg/dl)		5.0–7.2 mmol/l (90–130 mg/dl)
Peak postprandial			< 10.0 mmol/l (< 180 mg/dl)
Self-monitored blood glucose:			
Fasting/preprandial	4.0–5.0 mmol/l (70–90 mg/dl)		
Postprandial	4.0–7.5 mmol/l (70–135 mg/dl)		
Blood pressure	< 130/80 mmHg	< 130/80 mmHg (<125/75 when there is proteinuria)	< 130/80 mmHg
Total cholesterol	< 4.5 mmol/l (175 mg/dl)	< 5.0 mmol/l	
LDL-cholesterol	< 2.5 mmol/l (100 mg/dl)	< 3.0 mmol/l (115 mg/dl)	< 2.6 mmol/l (100 mg/dl)
HDL-cholesterol			> 1.1 mmol/l (40 mg/dl)
Triglycerides			< 1.7 mmol/l (150 mg/dl)

* For patients at significant risk of macrovascular complications

Appendix 4 – Useful addresses and websites

Societies and associations

Europe

European Association for the Study of Diabetes
Rheindorfer Weg 3
D-40591 Düsseldorf
Germany
Tel: +49 211 75 84 690
Fax: +49 211 75 84 69 29

European Atherosclerosis Society
Secretary: Professor Sebastiano Calandra
Sezione di Patologia GeneraleDipartimento di Scienze BiomedicheUniversita di Modena e Reggio Emilia
Via Campi 287
I-41100 Modena
Italy
Tel: +39 059 2055 423 (direct);
+39 059 2055 416/432/435 (labs)
Fax: +39 059 2055 426
Website: http://www.eas-society.org

European Heart Network
Rue Montoyer 31
B-1000 Brussels
Belgium
Tel: +32 2 512 9174
Fax: +32 2 503 3525
e-mail: ehn@skynet.be
Website: http://www-ehnheart.org

European Society of Cardiology
The European Heart House
2035 Route des Colles
B.P. 179 - Les Templiers
FR-06903 Sophia Antipolis
France
Tel : +33 4 92 94 76 00
Fax : +33 4 92 94 76 01
e-mail: webmaster@escardio.org
Website: http://www.escardio.org

Euopean Society of Hypertension
Website: http://www.eshonline.org

UK

British Cardiac Society
9 Fitzroy Square
London W1T 5HW
Tel: +44 20 7383 3887
Fax: +44 20 7388 0903
Website: http://www.bcs.com

British Heart Foundation
14 Fitzhardinge Street
London W1H 6DH
Tel: 020 79350185
Fax: 020 7486 5820
Heart Information line: 0845 070 8070
Website: http://www.bhf.org.uk

American Heart Association
One North Franklin
Chicago, IL 60606-3421
USA
Tel: 312 422 3000
Website: http:// www.aha.org

American Society of Hypertension
148 Madison Avenue
New York, NY 10016
USA
Tel: 212 696 9099
Fax: 212 696 0711
e-mail: ash@ash-us.org
Website: http://www.ash-us.org

Index

*Note: Page numbers followed by "f" indicate figures; page numbers followed by "t" indicate tables. Main entries are in **bold**. This index is in letter-by-letter order whereby spaces and hyphens in main entries are excluded from the alphabetization process. **Abbreviations:** CHD = coronary heart disease; CVD = cardiovascular disease.*